Foundations for Health Improvement

The most important aspect of modern medicine is
unquestionably Public Health, embracing as it does the four
fundamental historical functions of the physician:

to heal, to know, to predict, to organise.

(MARTI-IBANEZ 1958)

Foundations for Health Improvement

Productive Epidemiological Public Health Research
1919–1998

A comparison of research output in the United Kingdom and
the United States of America, with analysis of the structural,
organisational and political influences

Walter W Holland
with the assistance of
Leon Gordis
and
Susie Stewart, J Michael O'Brien
and Frank-Peter Schelp

The Nuffield Trust
FOR RESEARCH AND POLICY
STUDIES IN HEALTH SERVICES

London: TSO

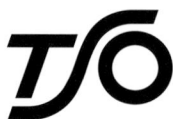

T∫O

Published by TSO (The Stationery Office) and available from:

Online
www.tso.co.uk/bookshop

Mail, Telephone, Fax & E-mail
TSO
PO Box 29, Norwich, NR3 1GN
Telephone orders/General enquiries: 0870 600 5522
Fax orders: 0870 600 5533
E-mail: book.orders@tso.co.uk
Textphone 0870 240 3701

TSO Shops
123 Kingsway, London, WC2B 6PQ
020 7242 6393 Fax 020 7242 6394
68-69 Bull Street, Birmingham B4 6AD
0121 236 9696 Fax 0121 236 9699
9-21 Princess Street, Manchester M60 8AS
0161 834 7201 Fax 0161 833 0634
16 Arthur Street, Belfast BT1 4GD
028 9023 8451 Fax 028 9023 5401
18-19 High Street, Cardiff CF10 1PT
029 2039 5548 Fax 029 2038 4347
71 Lothian Road, Edinburgh EH3 9AZ
0870 606 5566 Fax 0870 606 5588

TSO Accredited Agents
(see Yellow Pages)

and through good booksellers

First published 2002

ISBN 0117029947

Printed in the United Kingdom for The Stationery Office

ACKNOWLEDGEMENTS

This work would not have been possible without the help of many individuals in the US and the UK. This help has been invaluable in providing advice, information and opinions. The ultimate decisions, however, have been my own and I alone am responsible for what has been included or omitted.

In the United States, I am particularly grateful to Dr R Anderson, Dr L Breslow, Dr R Bulger, Dr G Comstock, Dr R Detels, Mr MK Gemmell, Mr F Karel, Dr Fitzhugh Mullen, Mr J Parascondola, Dr R Roemer and Mrs Lauren Le Roy.

In the UK, enormous help has been provided by Dr M Ashley-Miller, Dr G Draper, Dr P Ellwood, Professor C du V Florey, Professor P Hennessy, Mr P Holland, Professor G Knox, Professor D Miller, Dr E Mossialos, Professor J Pemberton, Mr C Webster and Dr B Williams.

I am most grateful to Claire Bird for her ability to decipher my handwriting and to Anna Maresso and Deme Nicolaou for their unfailing helpfulness on many occasions, particularly when I had difficulties with my computer. Last but not least, Fiona Holland provided encouragement and support throughout.

This work has been supported by the Nuffield Trust to whom I am grateful, in particular John Wyn Owen, Max Lehmann, Robert McIndoe and Patricia McKellar.

Contents

Preface

Foundations for Health Improvement is a further Nuffield Trust contribution to improving the health of the people of the United Kingdom. As the text illustrates, after 1945 the Nuffield Provincial Hospitals Trust, forerunner of the Nuffield Trust for Research and Policy Studies in Health Services, played a crucial role in the development and strengthening of epidemiological public health research. The Trust provided funds for the foundation of the Chairs in Social Medicine at the Universities of Oxford and Birmingham and has continued, without interruption, to promote epidemiological public health research for over fifty years. Although the sums of money available for disbursement have never been great, they have been used imaginatively as a catalyst to foster epidemiological public health research.

In 1999 the Nuffield Trust awarded a grant to Professor Walter Holland to look at productive public health research and what is needed to support it. The intention was to examine the conditions that promote good epidemiological public health by comparing the output of such research at different time periods in different countries, principally focusing on the United States and the United Kingdom in three time periods: 1918–1939, 1946–1970 and since 1970. Differences in the type, quality and advances in research in these countries were found during the specified time periods and this monograph analyses and compares these with individual, institutional and governmental policies as well as the contribution of various endowments.

Public Health: The Vision and the Challenge, Walter Holland's 1997 Rock Carling monograph, makes it clear that the knowledge base for the development of epidemiology and public health progressed at different rates and at different times in the UK and the US. It seemed that UK research was not as searching or as productive as US research between the two World Wars – 1919–1939 – but more relevant research, of better quality, was carried out in the UK than in the US after the end of World War II and up to about 1970. Since that time progress in the two countries has not shown such a contrast. *Foundations for Health Improvement* documents this and Professor Holland contends that, if anything,

UK research has shown a decline in quality while US research has improved. One of the aims of this analysis of the history of public health research in the US and the UK was to identify the major pieces of epidemiological public health research in the two nations that have improved our knowledge so that better health policies can be applied. This has been achieved.

Looking to the future, there are lessons to be learned to help us address some of the forthcoming challenges: the impact of globalisation on the determinants of national health; the policy issues around confidentiality; and the need for appropriate national, European and international public health law. Epidemiological public health research is an important area in terms of improving the health of populations and thus, ultimately, of individuals. History points to the importance of adequate resources and institutional frameworks to enable multidisciplinary work to be fostered as well as research support for the professions responsible for providing health services. Equally important is the contribution of society's interest in the political issues surrounding the health of the people. Of fundamental importance are the twin imperatives of independence and freedom to enquire and to publish findings. Professor Holland and his colleagues demonstrate that one of the lessons the past has shown is the need for epidemiological public health research to enable us to ask questions and to tackle problems which may not sit comfortably with politics or industry. With the developments in laboratory sciences, molecular technology, mathematics, statistics and computing there is a danger that epidemiological public health research is already far more interested in the analysis of micro-mechanisms and processes and less attuned to examining the macro problems and the solutions that are going to have to be developed to respond to and tackle issues of health inequality or ineffective health services. Investigation of mechanisms and processes, as Professor Holland reminds us, is reminiscent of the preponderance of laboratory research between the wars in the UK. To practitioners this is far less threatening and far more likely to lead to immediate rewards than tackling the macro problems. The need to undertake epidemiological field studies rather than relying only on routinely collected data, if important questions are to be addressed is emphasised. It is now crucial, however, that epidemiological public health research, which has a superlative record of achievement on both sides of the Atlantic in improving the health of people, does not lose its way or compromise but that it focuses instead on the relevant and sometimes unpopular questions effectively and with scientific rigour. After all, epidemiology and biostatistics, as analytical methods, are the foundation of scientific enquiry. The primary science of public health, directed towards an understanding of risk, injury and disease and concerned with populations rather than with individuals, separates it from the rest of medicine and constitutes the basic science of public health, which can help develop whole system strategies that reduce the underlying causes that make diseases common in populations.

John Wyn Owen CB
Secretary, Nuffield Trust

1. Introduction

During the eighteenth and nineteenth centuries major advances in public health were made in both the United Kingdom and the United States. The most important influences on changes in practice and conditions were the perceptions and observations of some individuals in authority of what was wrong and how things could be improved.

In spite of such historical landmarks as the Bills of Mortality, collected in London in the seventeenth century, systematic observations, proper collection of data and data analysis really only began in the middle of the nineteenth century. The basis for the systematic use of epidemiological investigation in outbreaks of disease was laid by John Snow in his study of cholera, William Farr in his collection of demographic and mortality data, and John Simon in his use of these investigations and others to improve public health practice in the United Kingdom. Similar heroes can be identified in the United States. Dorothy Porter[1] and Elizabeth Fee[2] provide excellent descriptions of how public health knowledge was developed and used on both sides of the Atlantic.

During the preparation of the book *Public Health: the Vision and the Challenge,*[3] it became clear that the knowledge base for the development of epidemiology and public health had progressed at different rates at different times in the UK and the US. Thus it seemed that UK research was not as searching or productive as US research between the two World Wars (1919–1939). Both the quantity and the quality of relevant research carried out, however, was greater in the UK after the end of World War II than in the US up to about 1970. Since that time, progress in the two countries has not shown such a contrast – if anything, UK research has shown a decline in quality while US research has improved.

A number of studies of research funding and organisation have compared practice between the two countries[4] and commented on practice in the UK[5-8] and the US.[9,10] Most of these studies have been carried out by people outwith the field who have not made any attempt at systematic assessment of either the research done or its quality. The present author (WWH) has been actively engaged in epidemiological public health research (EPHR), has been involved in a variety of research assessment and review activities and has an interest in the promotion of EPHR and the optimal conditions for its pursuit.

The first task, in chapters 2 and 3, was to describe the research done as comprehensively as possible. For the United Kingdom two methods were used. In the first period (1919–1939), the main journals were hand searched and, in addition, relevant catalogues and lists of publications for a number of bodies (for example, the Medical Research Council (MRC) and the Ministry of Health) were examined as well as books on the subject published during the period. Microbiological journals were excluded deliberately because any papers of public health significance in these were invariably referred to in the more general journals or in public health publications.

Each publication identified as relevant to EPHR was examined for content, method and application. A personal judgment was made as to its quality and relevance to public health, and publications considered to have met these two criteria are referred to in chapter 2.

This method does of course depend on the subjective opinion of one person (i.e. WWH). Publications may have been missed or wrongly evaluated. Within available resources, however, it was simply not possible to have all publications reviewed more than once or by more than one observer. And any form of quantitative assessment was not possible in the absence of a comprehensive database.

Some check of the validity of the identification of relevant publications was possible. Study of editorials, commentaries and book reviews in the *Lancet* and the *British Medical Journal* provided some check on whether important publications had been included, as did examination of the Medical Annuals, which are reviews of work done in the previous year. Chapter 2 was also reviewed by a number of expert colleagues who provided comments both on completeness and on the assessments made. In the final analysis, however, I am solely responsible for the judgments made.

For the period 1945–1998 (chapter 3) a different method of assessment was used. Systematic search of journals would have been an impossible task, because of both the increase in the number of relevant journals and the corresponding increase in the number of publications. In this period, therefore, I compiled a list of major topics and the most productive and influential authors and identified and read relevant and illustrative publications. My credentials for this task included my experience as a researcher during the period, my activities as an expert reviewer of a large number of publications, my editorship of the *International Journal of Epidemiology* and the *Oxford Textbook of Public Health*, and my membership of a number of editorial committees. I also convened a group of leading UK researchers who were invited to compile similar lists of topics and authors. The topics and authors identified were the result of consensus between the members of this group as described in the appendix to chapter 3.

No formal method of scoring was applied in these assessments and it was not considered appropriate to use formal criteria judgments in each subject or publication. In almost any EPHR publication, faults in design, execution or analysis can be identified. Different individuals will place more or less emphasis on one or other type of "failure". A formal method of assessment would have been a monumental task impossible within the resource constraints of this exercise and would not necessarily have improved the judgments made.

Similar methods were used for the analysis of EPHR in the two time periods in the United States. The task there was in many ways more complex in view of the enormous number of publications, research groups, institutions and funding bodies in the US. On the other hand, the analysis was helped by the existence of more symposia, research reviews and historical descriptions of research than exist in the UK. I also depended on the help of a number of American colleagues who identified work they considered as important. In addition, the records of the American Epidemiological Society helped to confirm the attribution of importance to individuals and work done. This Society, founded in 1927, is composed of a small group of senior epidemiologists who meet annually. Until the mid- to late 1960s, it was considered to be the most prestigious forum for the discussions of EPHR.[11,12]

Since the quantity of American EPHR was far greater than that carried out in the UK at all time periods, only the most important US work is cited.

The ultimate aim in chapters 2 and 3 was to identify the major pieces of EPHR in the UK and the US which have improved our knowledge so that better health policies can be applied. The major criterion was to identify EPHR work which led to the development and application of better public health policies. Thus methodological papers were only included if they resulted in a clear advance in the application of the findings – for example, the randomised controlled trial. Although the work may be open to criticism because of its unavoidably subjective nature, reviewers have agreed with the judgments made and I am, therefore, reasonably satisfied with the value system used.

Chapter 4 describes the structure, organisation and funding of public health research in the two countries between 1919 and 1998/9, while chapter 5 covers the main concerns of politics and society over the same period. Chapter 6 summarises the main trends and findings in research in the last century and looks at factors influencing both the quantity and the quality of EPHR. The concluding chapter attempts to synthesise these findings and suggest some possible reasons for the variability of research output. The annexes – a description of the types of research carried out in the former German Democratic Republic before and after the fall of the Berlin Wall (annexe 1) and a description of the investigation of BSE in the UK (annexe 2) – are intended to highlight, through two specific examples, the central importance of political expediency in EPHR.

The aim of the book as a whole is to provide an overview of epidemiological public health research in the twentieth century and to show how it has contributed to the making of health policy and to an improvement in health at a population level.

REFERENCES

1 Porter D. (1997) Public Health and centralization in the Victorian British State. In: *Oxford Textbook of Public Health*. 3rd edition. Detels R, Holland WW, McEwen J, Omenn GS (Eds). Vol. 1, pp 20–34.

2 Fee E. (1997) The origins and development of public health in the United States. In: *Oxford Textbook of Public Health*. 3rd edition. Detels R, Holland WW, McEwen J, Omenn GS (Eds). Vol. 1, pp 35–54.

3 Holland WW, Stewart S. (1998) *Public Health: The Vision and the Challenge.* London: Nuffield Trust.

4 Braun D. (1994) *Health Research and its Funding.* Country Reports, Vol. I Federal Republic of Germany and United States. Vol. II France and England. Federal Ministry for Research and Technology. Köln: DLR.

5 McLachlan G (Ed). (1971) *Portfolio for Health 1. The role and programme of the DHSS in health services research.* London: Nuffield Provincial Hospitals Trust.

6 McLachlan G (Ed). (1973) *Portfolio for Health 2. The developing programme of the DHSS in health services research.* London: Nuffield Provincial Hospitals Trust.

7 McLachlan G (Ed). (1978) *Five Years After. A review of health care management.* London: Nuffield Provincial Hospitals Trust.

8 House of Lords Select Committee on Science and Technology. (1988) *Priorities in Medical Research.* H L Paper 54–1. London: HMSO.

9 Institute of Medicine. (1997) *Linking Research and Public Health Practice: A review of CDC's programme of centres for research and demonstration of health promotion and disease prevention.* Washington DC: National Academy Press.

10 Institute of Medicine. (1988) *Committee for the study of the future of public health. Division of Health Care Services.* Washington DC: National Academy Press.

11 Paul JR. (1973) An account of the American Epidemiological Society. A retrospect of some 50 years. *Yale Journal of Biology and Medicine*, 46: 1–148.

12 Paul O. (1998) The last 25 years of the American Epidemiological Society: 1972–1996. *American Journal of Epidemiology*, 148: 104–130.

2. Epidemiological Public Health Research 1919–1939
The United Kingdom with Comparison to the United States

This chapter deals with epidemiological public health research (EPHR) in the inter-war period: firstly, and in more detail, in regard to the United Kingdom and then more briefly and selectively in the United States. The chapter is, therefore, split into two separate sections with references listed at the end of each part.

THE UNITED KINGDOM
As mentioned briefly in chapter 1, all relevant papers published in the *British Medical Journal (BMJ)*, *Lancet*, *Journal of Hygiene*, *Journal of the Royal Institute of Public Health (Journal of State Medicine)*, and *Medical Annual* were examined to determine the types and quality of EPHR carried out in the United Kingdom during this period. The Medical Research Council Special Report Series was also examined as well as Royal College of Physicians Reports and appropriate books and monographs. Editorials and comments in the *Lancet* and *BMJ* were a fruitful source of references and were useful in drawing attention to important issues and research findings that might otherwise have been overlooked. Journals of Bacteriology were not examined, on the grounds that any investigation of an epidemiological or public health nature would also be covered elsewhere.

We did not seek to describe exhaustively all the work done – much of it was descriptive, perhaps of one outbreak or one or two cases, and of variable quality. Relevant publications were examined to assess the degree of innovation of the findings, the quality of the methods of investigation and analysis, the conclusions, and the applicability of the findings to the health problems in this period.

This was necessarily a subjective analysis. The observations, however, were discussed with a number of appropriate colleagues to ensure that no important paper or finding had been omitted and there was a close match between the judgments of the author and others of those publications considered particularly relevant and good.

The volume and quality of medical research in general in this time period were limited. Academic medical research was only beginning to develop in the United Kingdom. The number of full-time university positions in medicine as a whole was very small, and in public health/epidemiology even smaller. Where a chair existed, the professor was often also the local Medical Officer of Health. Only in Scotland was there a tradition of a full-time academic position in public health.

The foundation of the London School of Hygiene in 1923–25 changed this position. As the *British Medical Journal* remarked on 17 March 1923 (page 477), "it is perfectly consonant with the psychology of the English race that the actual knowledge of preventive medicine and hygiene should be higher than its academic status…only in a minority of English universities can the doctorate be attained by proficiency in the subject! In some, ignorance of the principle of preventive medicine does not form a barrier to graduation". The editorial went on to emphasise that the aim must be to raise academic standards – but did not attempt to clarify how this might be done.

One month later (7 April) the *British Medical Journal* continued: "the fascination of good public health research has not even yet been properly appreciated". Concern with the standing, content and practice of public health and EPHR is confirmed in September (8 September, page 426) in an editorial on a recently published book on vital statistics from the United States. It criticises the book for the omission of epidemiology and mathematical theory, but is even more critical of practice in the UK and states that here the principles of vital statistics were not considered important in epidemiology and public health.

Sympathetic concern with EPHR is manifested by repeated reference to the publication of research findings, as well as to the progress of the London School of Hygiene.

The neglect of medical research generally in the period is, however, perhaps best described by Dr John Harman – himself a consultant physician at St Thomas' Hospital with a successful private practice and not an academic – in an editorial in the *British Medical Journal* in 1939 (page 339). In regretting the lack of research and experimental research in particular, he continues "we are still a nation of wealthy shopkeepers, whose health is looked after by clinicians as skilful in their craft as any in the world. Why should we waste money in research?" Harman then goes on to criticise this wrong-headed attitude.

Professional education in public health has been fully described by Acheson and Fee[1] and will not be considered here. Chapter 4 contains an outline of the staffing of academic public health in the UK. In this chapter we are concerned with the type of research done.

The major problems in this period were the result of communicable diseases, and it is, therefore, not surprising that most of the work published focused on these. Papers consisted usually of reports of outbreaks, control of specific diseases through the use of sera and other immunising agents, and towards the end of the period the results of treatment with some of the newly discovered chemotherapeutic agents (sulphanilamides). Several papers dealt with environmental factors such as housing, unemployment, poverty, and occupation. A number of studies were reported on the effect of deficiencies in nutrition – and the effect of supplementation of the diet. There were a few papers on chronic disease, particularly cancer – and some even on the effects of tobacco.

Discussion of many of the "expert" papers by senior figures – which either merely pontificate on their views of a disease, describe a few cases (with no denominator) or omit any numerical findings – has been omitted. A few of the papers concerned with EPHR in the Empire, particularly India and the Sudan, are considered if relevant.

Infectious / Communicable Disease Research
Studies on factors influencing the spread of infection, and thus their possible control, were undertaken by Topley and co-workers. This work was carried out in various locations, depending on where the main authors were employed, but the longest series of studies took place at the London School of Hygiene. Topley

was a bacteriologist, and not surprisingly, therefore, these studies were laboratory based, and considered as an example of experimental epidemiology. His co-workers in the later series of publications included the most eminent epidemiologist of the day, Professor Major Greenwood, and a future Professor of Medical Statistics, Austin Bradford Hill. The studies were all conducted on colonies of mice, and the favoured organism was ecteromelia. The Medical Research Council (MRC) was consistently a major funder of these investigations which, looked at with the benefit of hindsight, produced little knowledge useful in understanding either the behaviour of infections in man or their control. This is in contrast to the work of Pearl and Wade Hampton Frost in the United States. The conclusions drawn were general – that infective behaviour was variable, and that "artificial immunisation increased the resistance of mice to infection, but did not confer complete immunity, diet did not influence survival, and dispersal, or reducing the intimacy of contact may be effective in the early stages of the epidemic process in reducing the spread of infection".[2]

Descriptive studies of individual conditions were the most common and of very variable quality. There were many descriptions of influenza – for example, the spread of influenza in the industrial area of Halifax,[3] and the periodicity of "influenza".[4] But it was not until the influenza virus was isolated from ferrets, and transmission to man could be shown, that accurate serological methods of identification of the disease were devised.[5] The presumption of influenza being caused by a filterable virus was first advanced by Gibson and colleagues in a reputable series of animal experiments.[6]

There were a number of papers on encephalitis lethargica and other neurological infections which were well reviewed and summarised in a series of articles by McNalty.[7] Poliomyelitis merited some mention,[8] including a good description of a school outbreak,[9] but none were of the quality of US work done by Paul and his school at Yale.

Studies of measles and whooping cough were descriptive – usually of outbreaks in a town or village.[10] The denominator was often missing, except in the studies of Glover which were usually very thorough.[11] The prevention and control of measles, scarlet fever and diphtheria by the use of sera were reviewed and analysed, and recommendations made for their use in institutions and in the home.[12] An excellent analysis of how to maximise the effectiveness of passive convalescent serum immunisation for measles was made by Stocks.[13] An earlier paper on studies of outbreaks on ships was not as convincing.[14]

The investigations of streptococcal infection, particularly scarlet fever, puerperal fever and sore throats were of very variable quality.[15] Colebrook and colleagues[16,17] gave clear recommendations of feasible, effective measures for control. Studies of streptococcal disease were well carried out by Bradley[18,19] who nonetheless had great difficulty in getting support for his work from the Medical Research Council! The link between streptococcal disease and rheumatic disorders was considered by Glover as a result of his work on school outbreaks.[20] The relationship between dietary factors and immunity was largely experimental,[21] while others were concerned unsuccessfully with active immunisation against scarlet fever.[22]

Work on tuberculosis (TB) was not as frequent as might have been expected in view of its importance as a cause of disease at this time. Perhaps one of the wisest comments, made at the beginning of the period, was by Baskett:[23] "if a government concentrates on the question of real wages it does more to eliminate tubercle than it can do by any other means." The effectiveness of pasteurisation on elimination of the bovine TB bacillus in naturally infected milk was the subject of more than four years' experimental work at the National Institute of Research in Dairying. It was shown that pasteurisation at 62.8°C for 30 minutes did not "invariably" kill all TB bacilli, while 60°C for 20 minutes killed many – but left no safety margin.[24] About the same time, a good experimental study was published on the infectivity of milk from tuberculous cows and pasteurisation.[25] Wright[26] showed the efficacy of tuberculin tested (TT) milk and Newsholme[27] reviewed the problem of TB on the basis of a good vital statistical analysis of trends, age, sex, and geographical distribution. The "imperial interest" was demonstrated in an account of the effect of climate on TB in India. Rogers[28] used figures from jails because he considered this population to have accurate incidence rate figures – although he did not comment on such problems as selection, isolation, exposure and so on. Although there were a number of commentaries on BCG, particularly the Lübeck disaster, there were few other reasonable papers on epidemiology. Perhaps the only exceptions were on the frequency of TB in migrants from rural Essex to London in comparison to those who remained behind,[29] the importance of home contacts,[30] and the role of anthracosis, silicosis and TB in coal miners[31] – although this last paper was almost entirely on pathology and histology. Some years later a series of papers by D'Arcy Hart[32] dealt comprehensively with TB epidemiology in the "modern" manner.

The number of publications on the efficacy of immunisation, both passive and active, was surprisingly limited in view of the possibilities for control in the absence of effective forms of treatment. Work on diphtheria was mainly confined to laboratory studies,[33] or descriptions of experience in one place.[34]

Studies on the duration of passive immunity (14 days) to diphtheria were published after the availability of active immunisation.[35] Shortly thereafter a description of the progress of diphtheria prevention in London appeared,[36] although this was by no means the first such description.[37] The acceptability of diphtheria immunisation was investigated in schools in Edinburgh where Benson showed that only about half the children agreed to be immunised, but that the regime was effective and had no side-effects.[38] By contrast, a German author, Friedman,[39] commenting on infectious diseases in children in Berlin, reported that more than a million children had been immunised by 1928 with excellent results. Further articles on the effectiveness of diphtheria immunisation appeared in subsequent years.[40-44] A rare general article on the value of immunisation was based largely on experimental findings.[45]

In view of the frequency of reports of the use of immunising agents, both active and passive, it is perhaps surprising that the largest and longest series of experimental epidemiological studies by the most prestigious school (London School of Hygiene) and workers (Topley, Greenwood) never tackled the problem of the control of infectious disease in the long series of studies they did between 1922 and 1936.[3] These studies of the process of infection in mice colonies never investigated how the findings could be applied in the field to prevent the spread of infections or explored possible strategies using vaccines or other forms of immunisation for the prevention of disease.

Good epidemiological studies of outbreaks were carried out in schools by Allison Glover, who investigated the effect of age and ventilation on the spread of droplet infections in schools, as well as the arrangements of sleeping quarters and the consumption of pasteurised milk.[46] Similarly, Cruickshank examined the distribution and nature of food poisoning,[47] and Scott studied food poisoning due to eggs.[48] A Medical Officer of Health in Doncaster provided an excellent description of an outbreak of milk-borne scarlet fever and tonsillitis lasting 12 days where 27% of the 1343 persons at risk were infected (10% scarlet fever, 17% tonsillitis).[49] The Croydon typhoid epidemic of 1938 received mention, as did several outbreaks of dysentery in Glasgow[50] and Bedford.[51]

It is worth noting, in view of his later work, that Pickles published an account of an outbreak of catarrhal jaundice in Wensleydale in 1930[52] and Sonne dysentery in 1932.[53] Smallpox was still seen, for example, on Merseyside.[54] The aerial spread of streptococcal infections was analysed by Robert Cruickshank, a future professor of microbiology at St Mary's and at Edinburgh, and George Godber, a future Chief Medical Officer (CMO).[55]

Occupational and Industrial Factors

As has already been mentioned, this was an era of high unemployment. It is, therefore, not surprising that there were a number of publications on the relationship between employment and health. One of the most noteworthy publications was by Professor Major Greenwood who undertook a historical review by examining standardised mortality ratios (SMRs) in different occupations in comparison with that of the clergy.[56] His particular concern was with the control of juvenile employment and its harmful effects. Bradford Hill analysed the health of cotton operatives and showed how localised exhaust systems and vacuum stripping had improved conditions.[57] Recognition of byssinosis only came very much later. The problems of pneumoconiosis in coal miners was addressed in a descriptive study by Cummins of Cardiff.[58]

The prevention of industrial accidents was considered by looking at the experience in munitions factories during the war.[59] The prime causes were considered to be alcohol, carelessness, temperature in the workplace, ventilation and expected speed of production. Lane dealt with the prevention of lead poisoning or plumbism.[60] There was a series of general articles, reviews and editorials on the prevention of disease in industry – for example, respiratory disease in cotton operatives[61] – but a dearth of good epidemiological investigations.

A noteworthy paper by Lewis Fanning of the Medical Research Council looked at the problem of health (mortality) in the depressed areas.[62] In contrast to the findings of the report by Newman in his CMO's Annual Reports,[63] he wrote "there is no evidence from the trend of mortality rates from all causes of death that the health of the population of the distressed areas has been unfavourably affected by economic depression. Excessive mortality these areas have, but this is not peculiar to the year of depression. It has been a consistent feature of their mortality for at least the past 20 years. The existence of evil conditions is not mitigated by reason of their always having been evil". It is somewhat surprising that this forthright statement evoked no comment in the editorial pages, nor any subsequent correspondence.

By contrast there were one or two papers and reviews of the effects of overtime on health, and most remarkably, few or no papers investigating occupational hazards by epidemiological studies. Instead, investigations were done on animals, for example mineral oils in mice,[64] to determine the relation of oils to scrotal cancer. This is not unusual for the time in view of the paramountcy of pathology and Koch's postulates.

Nutrition and Nutritional Factors

Research into the effects of nutrition and nutritional constituents was important and common. The main topics covered were vitamins (and similar essential elements), the effect of nutrition on health generally and growth in particular, and the beneficial effects of milk and of iron on specific groups such as children and pregnant mothers.

Vitamins and "Accessory" Factors

There were innumerable studies on the role of vitamins in health. This was the era in which biochemists dominated the field, and it is, therefore, not surprising that most studies were laboratory based, linked to physiology, often done on animals or, if referring to humans, usually individual case studies or based on a small number of individuals or patients.

The scene was set by Gowland Hopkins who described a large number of laboratory, animal and physiological studies.[65] A remarkably prolific investigator, supported by the Medical Research Council and the Lister Institute, was Harriet Chick who was particularly notable for her work on the effect of vitamins A, C and D on children suffering from deprivation in Vienna in the early 1920s.[66-69]

A more epidemiological approach was followed by McCarrison in his ecological studies of beriberi and rice consumption in India. Interestingly he included animals, and birds in particular, in his observations.[70]

Experiments in man (and animals) were common – for example, the value of cod liver oil in the treatment of rickets.[71] The value of vitamins as anti-infective agents was investigated by Mellanby, who showed that in animals with vitamin A deficiency, death from sepsis was common.[72] In the same year Lady May Mellanby showed that vitamin D could prevent caries in children.[73] It is of interest in relation to the methods in use at that time that this experimental study was carried out on three groups of children numbering 23, 24 and 24. There was no matching and no randomisation. The standard of work (and view of epidemiology in the UK) is perhaps exemplified by a study of an outbreak of pellagra in a South African prison which states that it was caused by protein deficiency and reflects Goldberger's findings – a wrong interpretation of his work![74]

The role of nutrition in the aetiology of goitre in India was described by McCarrison. His epidemiological studies led him, however, to conclude that iodine deficiency was not the cause but merely a symptom of an underlying deficiency in metabolism. The cause, he maintained, was polluted water.[75]

In contrast to these largely biochemical, laboratory-based studies was the work of Sutherland, an Assistant Medical Officer in Aberdeenshire. He did a field experiment in which vitamins A and D were added to the diet of 294 school children whose rates of growth and resistance to infection were then compared to 281 control children from the same areas. This was not a proper randomised controlled trial but it was well designed and avoided some of the common pitfalls. Sutherland did not show any difference in growth or illness rates between the two groups, but the rest of the diet was unaffected and he concluded that this was more important in influencing growth and disease incidence.[76]

Finally, in this category of vitamins and other accessory factors, there were two major reviews by Gowland Hopkins[77] and Harris,[78] Director of the Medical Research Council Dunn Nutrition Unit in Cambridge.

Diet, Health and Growth

The studies of the effect of diet on health and growth were varied, ranging from pure epidemiological studies, such as those of Bradford Hill on a number of population groups, through detailed dietary studies by a nutritional scientist, such as Boyd Orr, and EPHR studies by medical officers of health – for example, M'Gonigle – to experimental studies, partly on animals.

A good example was an early study by Bradford Hill,[79] in which he showed that the rural workers were underfed (compared to the norms), although three-quarters of their income was spent on food (one-third on bread and flour). Nonetheless, the rural diet compared favourably with the diet of urban workers who had a higher income but spent less (relatively) on food, but more on meat and fats than rural dwellers. He found no evidence of malnutrition in the rural areas and no slowing of growth in rural children. An unusual component of this good study was an experiment on the health of mice fed on different diets, with the physiologist Leonard Hill.

In the previous year, Boyd Orr published a review on diet and public health, with particular reference to the importance of mineral elements in the maintenance of health,[80,81] while May Mellanby reviewed the effect of diet on dental health.[82] The importance of a "good" diet (based on experimental work in dogs on the production of calcified teeth), in an experimental study on the incidence of caries, was also published in the same year.[78]

An interesting study from the Public Health Department of Glasgow looked at growth and nutrition in slum children and found no correlation with quality of housing.[83] Boyd Orr, in an experimental-observational study in seven towns in Scotland, showed that the addition of milk to the diet of school children improved their health and increased rates of growth.[80] Later, he described the inadequate diets of 607 families in seven towns in Scotland.[84] His landmark study on food consumption in the UK showed the variations in diet between different social class groups and demonstrated the beneficial effects of a good diet on health and growth.[85] The importance of this survey was acknowledged by Lord Woolton after World War II and was used in designing a national food policy. The *British Medical Journal* also emphasised its importance in an editorial in 1936.[86]

M'Gonigle, Medical Officer of Health in Stockton-on-Tees, was another prolific worker on the effect of poverty on diet and ill-health.[87–89] One of his first papers, using only routine records, showed that the health of the mother and her efficiency have an important effect, independent of overcrowding and family size.

Perhaps one of the best studies on the importance of milk was also carried out by Boyd Orr.[90] In this, children in nine centres in three age groups were divided into four experimental groups – controls, additional biscuit, separated milk and whole milk. There were 40–50 children in each group and those given whole milk increased in both height and weight by about 20%.

Iron
Iron was another dietary component which was investigated in some depth, particularly in relation to anaemia. One of the most thorough surveys was carried out in Aberdeen.[91] The method of absorption and effect of iron was measured experimentally in 63 men and 68 women by Widdowson and McCance.[92] They did not find any relationship between "available" iron in the diet and haemoglobin. Of particular concern was that, in women with low haemoglobin, its level could not be raised by iron. In another study from Aberdeen, the problem of anaemia in pregnancy was shown to be particularly important in deprived women.[93] In a later study, Reid and Mackintosh were unable to detect reliably any long-term effect of anaemia during pregnancy.[94]

General Nutritional Study
An interesting study of the effect of diet in the prevention of disease looked at the particular effect of vitamin A – before the advent of chemotherapy or the recognition of the importance of strep infection. Five hundred and fifty women were included in an experiment in which vitamin A was given to alternate women. The authors found some protective effect, but did not discuss the problems of the design of the study in the interpretation of the results.[95]

Mortality and Morbidity
There were a number of interesting and reputable studies on various subjects related to chronic diseases and general mortality and morbidity.

General Mortality

Although the journals regularly reported on levels and trends of mortality, there were few good analytical studies. Of these, possibly the most noteworthy was carried out by Kermack and his colleagues to compare trends in Great Britain and Sweden between 1845 and 1930. The published report emphasised the importance of environment and infant mortality on the variations found.[96]

Infant and Neonatal Mortality

The relationship of infant mortality and economic status was dealt with somewhat superficially by comparison of trends between areas.[97] A somewhat better analysis of neonatal mortality had been carried out earlier by Newsholme who examined factors such as age (of mother), time, sex, causes, ante- and post-natal care and availability of midwifery services.[98]

Maternal Mortality

Several good investigations were reported. Munro and MacLennan's study, for example, demonstrated the importance of antenatal care and reported that about 10% of women were moribund by the time they arrived in hospital.[99] In another study of 20 000 cases, Munro and Sharman had previously established the role of pyrexia and infection in maternal mortality and had discussed the problem of antenatal care.[100] And the following year, Browne discussed the implications of these and other findings.[101] It is mainly on these studies that the confidential enquiries of maternal mortality – first instituted shortly after publication of these results – are based.

Weather and Disease

The role of weather and climate on disease was a subject investigated in particular by two researchers. Young at the National Institute of Medical Research first published a paper looking at mortality in children in a number of English towns between 1854 and 1919 and showed, in particular, the effect of cold in the preceding week.[102] The other researcher was Russell. An early example of his work on the effect of fog on respiratory disease showed that fog only affected mortality in the presence of low temperatures.[103] In a later analysis of time trends, he showed the independent effects of fog and low temperature. [104] The effect of weather on tuberculosis was investigated and an association was found between incidence and rain.[105] In a comprehensive analysis of the incidence of respiratory diseases, including pneumonia, Woods described both the magnitude of the problem in terms of mortality, the occurrence of epidemics, and the effects of climate, temperature, season, fog and geography.[106]

Cancer

There were a number of studies on the epidemiology of cancer, although most were experimental, often carried out on animals.[107-111] None of these studies, however, involved an adequate epidemiological design – all followed the then current preoccupation with animal exposure and experimentation.

The later studies by the Kennaways from the Royal Cancer Hospital on cancer of the lung, larynx and bladder followed a more adequate epidemiological approach.[112-113] Their paper on cancer of the bladder was one of the first to develop methods of analysis of occupational risks, still used today.

Tobacco

Tobacco as a possible health hazard was the subject of a major lecture by one of the leading physicians of the time although cancer of the lung was not considered.[114] The composition of cigarettes, and the possibility of "denicotinised tobacco" was considered by Dixon in 1927.[115] The first study identified on the role of tobacco and cancer was published in 1932 by the University of Birmingham at the request of the British Empire Cancer Campaign.[116] Interest had apparently been aroused by the high incidence of cancer of the lung in workers in the tobacco manufacturing industries. The study showed the production of cancer-inducing agents by the combustion of tobacco in mice. The (unidentifiable) authors concluded that the high incidence was caused by the dust in the tobacco factories! A few years later a study on 40 cases of duodenal ulcer (DU) and 400 controls showed a slight excess of DU in smokers, which became very marked if they inhaled.[117] None of these papers referred to the findings in Germany of an association between cancer of the lung and smoking, which were beginning to appear.

Other Chronic Diseases

Reasonable studies on specific conditions began to appear towards the end of this period. Examples included the trend in mortality for pernicious anaemia with the introduction of effective therapy,[118] and on diabetes.[119] Factors influencing the occurrence of asthma were studied by Fraenkel, a refugee from Germany, who compared his findings in the UK with those in Germany,[120] while Bedson published an excellent account of an outbreak of psittacosis in the London Zoo. [121]

Conclusion

In the 20 years under review in this chapter, quite a number of investigations relevant to EPHR were undertaken and published, most of them concerned with infectious disease. The studies referenced are those considered to have value, being both relevant to the problems of the day, and reasonable methodologically.

Three comments are relevant here. Firstly, a number of researchers who became prominent in later years were already publishing good studies at this time, – perhaps the best example of this is Austin Bradford Hill, although for whatever reasons, not all his publications during this time period were of equal merit.

Secondly, it is surprising how few of the leading figures of the day were publishing critical analyses either of other researchers' findings or of the methods in common use. Their studies were mainly descriptive, philosophical or historical. Self-criticism or the mention of possible deficiencies in an investigation were relatively rare. The one exception – which may reveal my own biases – were the papers of Bradford Hill which were invariably cautious in their interpretation.

Thirdly, there was a dearth of good studies on the control of disease – with the exception of the studies of puerperal fever.

In spite of these observations made with the benefit of hindsight, it is surprising how many editorials, commentaries and notes published in the *British Medical Journal*, *Lancet* and other journals, including the *Medical Annual*, commented and referred to the importance of public health and prevention. The congratulatory editorials on the foundation of the London School of Hygiene, and the condemnation of the lack of concern for these specialities in medical education are prime examples of this. But also striking was that both the *British Medical Journal* and the *Lancet* not infrequently reported on the Annual Public Health Reports of individual Medical Officers for Health, and not only on that of the Chief Medical Officer. In spite of considerable sympathy for the subject, however, EPHR was not prolific in this period.

REFERENCES

1 Fee E, Acheson RM (Eds). (1991) *A History of Education in Public Health*.
London: Oxford University Press.

2 Greenwood M, Bradford Hill A, Topley WWC, Wilson J. (1936) *Experimental
Epidemiology*. Medical Research Council Special Report Series
No. 209. London: Medical Research Council.

3 Garvie A. (1919) The Spread of Influenza in an Industrial Area. *British
Medical Journal*, 2: 519–523.

4 Spear BE. (1934) The Periodicity of Influenza. *Lancet*, 2: 1331–1333.

5 Laidlaw PP. (1935) Influenza a Virus Disease. *Lancet*, 2: 1118–1124.

6 Gibson G, Bowman FB, Connor JI. (1919) Influenza, a Filterable Virus?
British Medical Journal, 1: 331–335.

7 McNalty AS. (1925) Epidemic Diseases of the Central Nervous System.
Lancet, 1: 475–480; 532–537; 594–599.

8 Kinneir Wilson SA. (1928) Aetiology and Treatment of Acute Poliomyelitis.
Lancet, 1: 11–14.

9 Scott Brown WG. (1931) An Epidemic of Bulbar Type of Poliomyelitis. *Lancet*,
2: 1287–1293.

10 Halliday JL. (1928) *The Spread of Measles*. MRC Special Report Series
No. 120. London: Medical Research Council.

11 Glover JA. (1928) Nasopharyngeal Epidemics in Public Schools. *British
Medical Journal*, 2: 87–91.

12 Nabarro DN, Signy AG. (1931), Prevention and Control of Measles,
Scarlet Fever, and Diphtheria in Institutions and the Home. *British Medical
Journal*, 2: 599–603.

13 Stocks P. (1931) Some Observations on the Control of Measles Epidemics. *British Medical Journal*, 2: 977–980.

14 Dudley SF. (1924) Fundamental Factors Concerned in the Spread of Infectious Diseases. *Lancet*, 1: 1141–1146.

15 Riddell J. (1934) Epidemiology of Scarlet Fever in a Landward Area. *British Medical Journal*, 1: 276–278.

16 Colebrook L. (1933) Puerperal Fever: Its Aetiology and Prevention. *British Medical Journal*, 2: 723–726.

17 Paine CG. (1935) Aetiology of Puerperal Infection with Special Reference to Droplet Infection. *British Medical Journal*, 1: 243–246.

18 Bradley WH. (1938) The Spread of Streptococcal Disease. *British Medical Journal*, 2: 733–738.

19 Hobson FG. (1938) The Conduct of a School Epidemic. *British Medical Journal*, 2:171–175.

20 Glover JA. (1930) Incidence of Rheumatic Diseases. *Lancet*, 1: 499–505; 607–612; 733–738.

21 Burton AHG, Balmain AR. (1930) Vitamin A and strep anti toxic immunity. *Lancet*, 1: 1.

22 Benson WT, Rankine K. (1934) Active Immunisation Against Scarlet Fever. *Lancet*, 2: 1181–1185.

23 Baskett BGM. (1920) Public Health Versus the State. *British Medical Journal*, 1: 44.

24 Meanwell LJ. (1927) An Investigation of Pasteurisation on the Bovine TB Bacillus in Naturally Infected Milk. *Journal of Hygiene*, 26: 392–402.

25 White, RG. (1926) Study of the Effect of Pasteurisation on the Infectivity of Milk of Tuberculous Cows. *Lancet*, 1: 222–226.

26 Wright NC. (1929) Incidence of TB Infection in Milk Supplies of Scottish Cities. *British Medical Journal*, 2: 452–454.

27 Newsholme A. (1926) The Present Position of the TB Problem. *Lancet*, 1: 1021–1026.

28 Rogers L. (1925) TB Incidence and Climate in India. *British Medical Journal*, 1: 256–259.

29 Bradford Hill A. (1925) *Internal Migration and its Effect upon Death Rates; with Special Reference to the County of Essex*, London: Medical Research Council Special Report Series.

30 Kayne GG. (1935) TB in Home Contacts, Incidence and Contagion. *British Medical Journal*, 1: 692–696.

31 Cummins SL. (1931) Athracosis, Silicosis, and TB in Coal Miners. *Lancet*: 1: 235–238.

32 D'Arcy Hart PM. (1937) Prevention of Pulmonary TB Among Adults in England. *Lancet*, 1: 969–973; 1033–1035; 1093–1100.

33 Glenny T. (1925) Principles of Immunity Applied to Protective Inoculation against Diphtheria. *Journal of Hygiene*, 24: 301–320.

34 Kinlock JP, Smith J, Taylor JS. (1927) Newer Knowledge of Diphtheria and Scarlet Fever and its Application to Hospital Practice and Community Immunisation. *Journal of Hygiene*, 26: 327–356.

35 Munro-Jones EG, Kershaw JD. (1933) Duration of Passive Immunity to Diphtheria. *British Medical Journal*, 2: 969–970.

36 Forbes JG. (1937) Progress of Diphtheria Prevention. *British Medical Journal*, 2: 1209–1213.

37 Hutt CW. (1925) Diphtheria Immunisation in a Metropolitan Borough. *Lancet*, 2: 962–965.

38 Benson WT. (1924) Diphtheria Prevention: The Schick Test and Active Immunisation in Various Schools and Institutions in Edinburgh. *Lancet*, 2: 949–955.

39 Friedman U. (1928) Epidemiology of Infectious Diseases . *Lancet*, 2: 211–217.

40 May PM, Dudley SF. (1932) Active Immunisation and Diphtheria. *Lancet*, 1: 172–173.

41 Burn M, Fellowes V. (1934) Diphtheria Immunisation. A Review of 8 Years' Work in Birmingham. *Lancet*, 2: 1181–1185.

42 Ashworth Underwood E. (1935) Immunisation Against Diphtheria by Means of a Single Dose of APT. *Lancet*, 1: 137–139.

43 Thomas DJ, Howell NG. (1935) Diphtheria Immunisation in Action. *Lancet*, 1: 579–581.

44 Parrish HJ, Wright J. (1935) Schick Test and Active Immunisation in Relation to Epidemic Diphtheria. *Lancet*, 1: 600–604.

45 McIntosh J. (1926) Prophylactic and Therapeutic Immunisation and its Interpretation. *Lancet*, 2: 889–892.

46 Glover JA. (1928) Nasopharyngeal Epidemics in Public Schools. *British Medical Journal*, 2: 87–91.

47 Cruickshank J. (1929) Distribution and Nature of Food Poisoning. *British Medical Journal*, 2: 443–446.

48 Scott WM. (1930) Food Poisoning due to Eggs. *British Medical Journal*, 2: 56–58.

49   Watson R. (1937) An Outbreak of Milk-Borne Scarlet Fever and Tonsillitis in Doncaster. *British Medical Journal*, 1: 1189–1193.

50   Block E. (1938) Glasgow Experience of Increased Dysentery Prevalence. *British Medical Journal*, 1: 836–839.

51   Bowes GK. Outbreak of Sonne Dysentery due to Milk. *British Medical Journal*, 1: 1092–1093.

52   Pickles WN. (1930) Epidemic Catarrhal Jaundice. *British Medical Journal*, 1: 944–946.

53   Pickles WN. (1932) Sonne Dysentery in a Yorkshire Dale. *Lancet*, 2: 31–32.

54   Hanna W. (1930) Note on the Outbreak of Smallpox in Merseyside. *Lancet*, 2: 990–991.

55   Cruickshank R, Godber GE. (1939) Aerial Spread of Streptococcal Infections. *Lancet*, 1: 741–746.

56   Greenwood M. (1922) Influence of Industrial Employment and Health. *British Medical Journal*, 2: 667–672; 752–758.

57   Bradford Hill A. (1930) *Health of Cotton Operatives*. London: MRC Industrial Health Research Board Publication No. 59.

58   Cummins SL. (1935) Pneumoconiosis with Special Reference to the Silico-Anthracosis of Coal Miners. *British Medical Journal*, 2: 286–290.

59   Vernon HM. (1919) Causation and Prevention of Industrial Accidents. *Lancet*, 1: 549–550.

60   Lane RE. (1936) The Prevention of Industrial Plumbism. *Lancet*, 2: 206–211.

61   Anon. (1936) Editorial on Respiratory Disease in the Cotton Industry. *Lancet*, 2: 67.

62 Lewis Fanning E. (1937) A Study of the Trend of Mortality Rates in Urban Communities of England and Wales with Specific Reference to Depressed Areas. *Lancet*, 1: 865–867.

63 Holland WW, Stewart S. (1998) *Public Health, the Vision and the Challenge.* London: Nuffield Tust.

64 Twortt CC, Ing HR. (1928) Mule Spinners Cancer and Mineral Oils. *Lancet*, 2: 752–754.

65 Hopkins GF. (1920) The Present Position of Vitamins in Clinical Medicine. *British Medical Journal*, 2: 147–160.

66 Chick H, Dalyell EJ. (1921) Influence of Foods Rich in Accessory Factors in Stimulating Development in Backward Children. *British Medical Journal*, 2: 1061–1066.

67 Chick H, Dalyell H, Hume M, et al. (1920) Clinical Study of Children in Vienna. *Lancet*, 2: 7–12.

68 Chick H. (1932) Relation of UV Light to Nutrition. *Lancet*, 2: 325–380; 377–384.

69 Chick H. (1923) Current Theories of the Aetiology of Pellagra. *Lancet*, 2: 341–346.

70 McCarrison R. (1924) Rice in Relation to Beriberi in India. *British Medical Journal*, 1: 414–420.

71 Wagner R, Winnberger H. (1924) Clinical Observations on the Value of Oxidised Cod Liver Oil in the Therapy of Rickets. *Lancet*, 2: 55–57.

72 Green HN, Mellanby E. (1928) Vitamin A as an Anti-Infective Agent. *British Medical Journal*, 2: 691–697.

73 Mellanby M, Pattison CL. (1928) Action of Vitamin D in Preventing the Spread and Promoting the Arrest of Caries in Children. *British Medical Journal*, 2: 1079–1082.

74 Wilson WH. (1930) Note on the Aetiology of Pellagra. *British Medical Journal*, 1: 101–103.

75 McCarrison R. (1933) Food and Goitre. *British Medical Journal*, 2: 671–675.

76 Sutherland R. (1934) Vitamins A and D: Relation to Growth and Resistance to Disease. *British Medical Journal*, 1: 791–795.

77 Hopkins GF. (1935) The Study of Human Nutrition, the Outlook Today. *British Medical Journal*, 1: 571–577.

78 Harris LJ. (1933). Significance of Vitamins in Practical Experience. *British Medical Journal*, 2: 367–373.

79 Bradford Hill A. (1925) Physiologic and Economic Study of the Diets of Workers in Rural Areas, Compared with those of Workers Resident in Urban Districts. *Journal of Hygiene*, 24: 189–240.

80 Orr JB. (1928) Milk Consumption and Growth in School Children. *Lancet*, 1: 202–203.

81 Orr JB. (1924) Diet and the Public Health. *British Medical Journal*, 2: 504–512.

82 Mellanby M, Pattison CL, Proud JW. (1924) Effect of Diet on Development and Extension of Caries in Teeth of Children. *British Medical Journal*, 2: 354–355.

83 Murray AMT. (1927) Growth and Nutrition of the Slum Child in Relation to Housing. *Journal of Hygiene*, 26: 198–203.

84 Orr JB, Clark ML. (1930) A Dietary Survey. *Lancet*, 2: 594–598.

85 Orr JB. (1936) *Food, Health and Income*. London: Macmillan.

86 Anon. (1936) Editorial on Nutritional Survey by Boyd Orr. *British Medical Journal*, 1: 587.

87 M'Gonigle GCM, McKinlay PL. (1932) An Investigation into the Effect of Certain Factors upon Child Health and Child Weight.
Journal of Hygiene, 32: 465–488.

88 M'Gonigle GCM, Kirby J. (1936) *Poverty and Public Health*. London: Victor Gollancz.

89 M'Gonigle GCM. (1933) Poverty, Nutrition and the Public Health.
Proceedings of the Royal Society of Medicine, 26, Part 1: 677–687.

90 Orr JB. (1928) Influence of Milk Consumption on Rate of Growth of Schoolchildren. *British Medical Journal*, 1: 140–141.

91 Davidson LSP, Fullerton HW, Howie JW, et al (1933) Nutrition in relation to anaemia. *British Medical Journal*, 1: 685–690.

92 Widdowson EM, McCance RA. (1936) Iron in Human Nutrition. *Journal of Hygiene*, 36: 13–23.

93 Fullerton HW. (1936) Anaemia in Poor Class Women, with Special Reference to Pregnancy and Menstruation. *British Medical Journal*, 2: 523–528.

94 Reid WJS, Mackintosh JM. (1937) Influence of Anaemia and Poor Social Circumstances During Pregnancy on a Subsequent History of Mother and Child. *Lancet*, 2: 1389–1392.

95 Green HN, Pinder D, Davis G, Mellanby E. (1931) Diet as a Prophylactic Agent Against Puerperal Sepsis. *British Medical Journal*, 2: 595–598.

96 Kermack WO, McKendrick AC, McKinlay PL. (1934) Death Rates in Great Britain and Sweden. Some General Regularities and their Significance. *Lancet*, 1: 698–703.

97 McKinlay PL. (1928) Infant Mortality and Economic Status. *Lancet*, 2: 938–940.

98   Newsholme A. (1920) Neonatal Mortality. *Lancet*, 1: 1097–1102.

99   Munro KJM, McLennan HR. (1932) An Investigation into the Mortality in Maternity Hospitals and the Influencing Factors. *Lancet*, 1: 633–637.

100   Munro KJM, Sharman A. (1931) An Investigation into Maternal Mortality and Mortality in the Domiciliary Services of Maternity Hospitals. *Lancet*, 2: 201–204.

101   Browne FJ. (1932) Antenatal Care and Maternal Mortality. *Lancet*, 2: 1–4.

102   Young M. (1924–1925) Influence of Weather Conditions on Mortality from Bronchitis and Pneumonia in Children. *Journal of Hygiene*, 23: 151–175.

103   Russell WT. (1924) The Influence of Fog on Mortality from Respiratory Diseases. *Lancet*, 2: 335–339.

104   Russell WT. (1926) The Relative Influence of Fog and Low Temperature. *Lancet*, 2: 1128–1130.

105   Gordon W, Ash WM. (1928) Rain-Bearing Winds and Early Phthisis in Derbyshire. *British Medical Journal*, 1: 337–339.

106   Woods HM. (1928) On the Statistical Epidemiology of Respiratory Diseases. *Lancet*, 1: 539–543.

107   Leitch A. (1923) Experimental Inquiry into the Causes of Cancer. *British Medical Journal*, 2: 1–7.

108   Kennaway EL. (1924) On the Cancer Producing Factor in Tar. *British Medical Journal*, 1: 564–567.

109   Twort CC, Ing HR. (1928) Mule Spinners' Cancer and Mineral Oils. *Lancet*, 1: 752–754.

110   Gye WG. (1925) The Aetiology of Malignant New Growths. *Lancet*, 1: 109–116.

111 Barnard JE. (1925) The Microscopical Examination of Filterable Viruses Associated with Malignant New Growths. *Lancet*, 1: 117–123.

112 Kennaway NM, Kennaway EL. (1936) A Study of the Incidence of Cancer of the Lung and Larynx. *Journal of Hygiene*, 36: 236–267.

113 Henry SA, Kennaway NM, Kennaway EL. (1931) Incidence of Cancer of the Bladder and Cancer of the Prostate in Certain Occupations. *Journal of Hygiene*, 31: 125–137.

114 Rolleston H. (1926) Medical Aspects of Tobacco. *Lancet*, 1: 961–965.

115 Dixon WE. (1927) The Tobacco Habit. *British Medical Journal*, 2: 719–725.

116 University of Birmingham. (1932) The Role of Tobacco Smoking in the Production of Cancer. *Journal of Hygiene*, 32: 293–300.

117 Trowell OA. (1934) Relation of Tobacco Smoking to the Incidence of Chronic DU. *Lancet*, 1: 808–809.

118 Bradford Hill A. (1935) Mortality from Pernicious Anaemia in England and Wales. *Lancet*, 1: 43–46.

119 Stocks P. (1935) Lengthening of Life by Modern Therapy in PA and Diabetes. *British Medical Journal*, 1: 1013–1017.

120 Fraenkel EM. (1938) Moulds and Asthma. *British Medical Journal*, 2: 68–69.

121 Troup AG, Adams R, Bedson SP. (1939) Outbreak of Psittacosis at the London Zoo. *British Medical Journal*, 1: 51–55.

THE UNITED STATES

This period was a formative time for epidemiology in the United States. Despite landmark studies, such as those carried out by Snow on cholera years before, the discipline was, in general, not well recognised or established and it often appeared to be taking a defensive posture in trying to legitimise itself. This thrust the newly developing discipline into the centre of the ongoing discussions of the relative values of so-called "basic" research as against those of "applied" research, exemplified by EPHR.

In the United States during this time, there was a significant growth in the numbers and size of schools of public health. The Rockefeller Foundation played a significant role in fostering this growth as well as in introducing Preventive Medicine into the curricula and departmental structures of medical schools. But it was mainly in schools of public health where epidemiology was able to grow and develop and where the foundations could be laid for its fundamental relationship to the development of public policy. Perhaps as a result, the relevance of epidemiology for clinical practice and clinical policy took longer than it should have done to be appreciated.

The period was one in which the role of the federal government in research was extremely limited. Most of the support came from private foundations. Although a one-room "laboratory of hygiene" was established by the federal government in 1887, it was not until 1938 that the federal role was expanded through grants to universities and other research organisations. This programme remained limited throughout World War II and only after that did it expand dramatically, having an extraordinary impact on medical and health-related research in the United States, including EPHR.

The development of epidemiological methods was crucial in establishing epidemiology as a scientific discipline in its own right. Since infectious diseases were the primary public health problem of the time, many of these advances were made in the context of research on these diseases. From about 1913, Wade Hampton Frost began to study the relation between water quality and disease. Frost began to define epidemiology and refine its methodology, particularly after he became the first chairman of the Department of Epidemiology at the Johns Hopkins School of Hygiene and Public Health – the first autonomous academic department of epidemiology in the world.[1–3] The very name of the School suggests the role of epidemiology and other scientific disciplines: the word "hygiene" denoted hygiene in the German sense – the science underlying the practice of public health. To this day the School continues to stress the need for both – not only the study of the professional practice of public health, but also the building of the scientific basis for public health practice and policy. Epidemiology was clearly the discipline most integral to this close relationship.

Mortality and Morbidity

Advances took place in the design of community surveys and in approaches to the analyses of morbidity and mortality data. The first morbidity survey based on an entire community was conducted by Sydenstricker in Hagerstown, Maryland from 1921–1924.[4,5]

In 1933 Frost encouraged the use of person-years in survival analysis.[6] Although he was probably not the first to use person-years, its use spread after he taught it to his students who used it in their studies. Frost proposed the concept of secondary attack rate in his paper, *The familial aggregation of infectious diseases*, published in 1938.[7] In the context of his interest in tuberculosis, he described the cohort phenomenon (1939),[8] pointing out the problems in interpreting trends based on cross-sectional data obtained at intervals over calendar time. His approach to the investigation of disease is exemplified by his study of diphtheria.[9]

Work intensified on the relationship of certain exposures to mortality and morbidity. For example, the J-shaped curve of alcohol and mortality was reported by Pearl in 1924.[10]

Infectious / Communicable Disease Research

These years saw a period of major contributions to our understanding of communicable diseases, particularly impressive since these advances were achieved in the absence of the knowledge and methods of modern molecular biology. The new knowledge included not only specific micro-organisms responsible for specific infectious diseases, but also a growing recognition that other factors above and beyond the organism itself were required for disease to result. Among the most outstanding epidemiological accomplishments were those of the Armed Forces Epidemiology Board. These represented an early integration of laboratory investigation with epidemiological studies. The grouping and typing of streptococci permitted the spread of streptococci to be characterised, and with the development of tests for type-specific antibodies, the knowledge gained of the epidemiology of the organism and its non-suppurative sequelae of rheumatic fever and glomerulonephritis was greatly enhanced. This information also permitted the study of penicillin treatment and the benefit of prophylaxis, using sites such as the Great Lakes Naval Station where a pattern of outbreaks after each arrival of susceptible new recruits had been clearly identified.[11] This knowledge was also used in the investigation of outbreaks.[12]

Maxcy's characterisation of Murine (endemic) Typhus represented a milestone in the use of epidemiology for elucidating the mode of transmission of a disease. In order to clarify the issue, Maxcy plotted the cases in Montgomery, Alabama and created a spot map on the basis of location of residence of each afflicted individual.[13] Spot maps were not new and had been used by Snow, and Maxcy found that the results plotted by residence were not particularly dramatic. When he plotted the cases by place of employment, however, a marked clustering was observed. He localised the cases to food processing plants and later *Rickettsia mooseri* was identified as the causal agent.

Occupational and Industrial Factors

Perhaps the first recognition of the healthy worker effect was that of Thompson in 1928.[14] He wrote: "The wide difference in the rate of respiratory sickness among those who quit compared with those who tend to remain in the industry suggests the existence of a process of selection of workers resulting from their reaction to given working conditions. Those susceptible to respiratory diseases apparently do not remain many years in a working environment for which they are not physically well suited."

Nutrition and Nutritional Factors

One set of classic studies of this era were Goldberger's studies of pellagra which led in 1920 to identification of niacin deficiency as the cause.[15] Goldberger and his colleagues conducted animal and human experiments, observational studies, and intervention studies. His major finding that family income and other economic factors correlated with pellagra incidence in seven cotton-mill villages of South Carolina in 1916 was crucial in clarifying the aetiology of the disease. He was able to refute the generally held belief that pellagra was caused by some as yet unidentified microorganism. In 1918, Warren and Sydenstricker wrote:[16]

"The effects on health when diet is reduced below physiological needs, in quantity or quality, are well known. The effects of inadequate or improperly balanced diet are factors in the causation of sickness which have been noted by practically all physicians and health workers. The recent findings of Goldberger show clearly that an unbalanced diet causes pellagra, a disease which is found more frequently in families with low incomes than among the well-to-do. Furthermore, while diet is not a specific factor in the causation of tuberculosis, as in pellagra, the undernourished prove easy victims to the tubercle bacillus."

Two important issues emerged from the work of Goldberger and others above and beyond the contribution to nutritional research. First, as cited by Winslow, [17] Goldberger's work was a demonstration of what has been termed the epidemiological transition from infectious to non-infectious (chronic) diseases with its important implications for public health practice. Second, this work emphasised the multifactorial nature of disease and the importance of social factors in the development of disease, even when a specific causation is known.

Clinical Trials

Perhaps the first clinical trial was that reported by Amberson and colleagues in 1931.[18] The first controlled trial of vaccination against tuberculosis was started in 1932 and reported by Wells in 1944.[19] Community trials in which communities rather than individuals are randomized were exemplified by the studies of fluoride and dental caries described below.[20–22]

Dental Epidemiology

Dental epidemiology was a prominent area of EPHR in the US during this period. It involved the development of measures of dental pathology; the development and first use of decayed, missing and filled (DMF) index for dental epidemiology studies was reported by Klein and colleagues in 1938.[23] Studies were conducted relating the DMF indices in different communities to the concentration of natural fluoride in their drinking water.[20,21] This led to the Kingston-Newburgh trial after World War II in which two comparable cities on the Hudson River in New York were selected for study. Since individuals could not be randomly assigned to source of drinking water, assignment was of community rather than of individual. The water in Newburgh was fluoridated and Kingston served as an unfluoridated control. Further evidence of a causal association was provided by communities which had introduced fluoridation and subsequently approved voter referenda to have fluoridation stopped. Such communities demonstrated the initial fall in DMF rates with fluoridation followed by subsequent increases in DMF rates when fluoridation was terminated.[22]

Tobacco

This period saw the beginnings of concern with smoking – perhaps the best example of this was the study by Pearl on the relationship of smoking to length of life.[24]

Cancer

During this time Pearl also published a famous paper on the relationship between cancer and tuberculosis.[25] He suggested, on the basis of post-mortems at Johns Hopkins of patients with cancer, that since there was a deficit of tuberculosis among these individuals, the latter protected against cancer. This paper has achieved fame as an illustration of the need for care in the choice of controls (and cases) in case-control studies. As has been pointed out on many occasions, this negative association could probably be explained by the fact that patients with tuberculosis and cancer were less likely to be admitted to Johns Hopkins than those with cancer alone. This fallacy has come to be associated with the name of Berkson[26] – a statistician at the Mayo Clinic who used the same argument in trying to refute the association of smoking with cancer of the lung.

Interest in the causes of cancer also began to develop during this period and the first attempts were made to apply EPHR methods to the study of cancer – for example, Gilliam.[27]

Health Care/Services

The interest in improving the provision of health services on the basis of scientific facts was first developed by Falk and his colleagues,[28] in the longitudinal investigations of disease and medical care. Sydenstricker became closely involved and concerned with the need to develop a sound health policy based on his studies of health insurance and health experience of workers. These are recounted by Falk.[29]

There were, of course, numerous other good EPHR studies carried out at this time. This section has, however, tried to highlight the outstanding contributions made in the US rather than to provide an exhaustive listing. Zinsser provides a valuable account of the major concerns.[30]

As can be seen, the number and importance of research studies was somewhat greater than in the UK at this time. In marked contrast to the UK, only one epidemiologist attempted to base his work on laboratory (experimental) studies[31] and he abandoned them rapidly, in contrast to Topley and his colleagues in the UK. Obviously the leadership of Falk, Frost, Goldberger, Maxcy, Pearl and Sydenstricker exerted a profound influence on the direction of EPHR in the USA. This was particularly evident at the Johns Hopkins School of Hygiene and Public Health as recounted by Fee.[32]

Conclusion

The years before World War II were characterised in the US by the emergence of epidemiology as a recognised discipline, by its contributions to a number of disease areas, particularly diseases of infectious origin, and by a transition as epidemiology began to be applied to chronic diseases. In the course of making these contributions, major advances in methodology were developed. Public health and consequently epidemiological research, however, were often seen as separate from medicine and medical research although attempts were made to reduce this tension.[33] Only after World War II, with the infusion of federal grant funds into medical research, did epidemiology grow with great rapidity and did its inter-relationships with medicine become accepted facts.

REFERENCES

1 Sartwell PE. (1976) The contribution of Wade Hampton Frost. *American Journal of Epidemiology*, 104: 386–391.

2 Maxcy KF. (1941) *Papers of Wade Hampton Frost: A contribution to Epidemiological Method.* New York: The Commonwealth Fund.

3 Stebbins EL. (1976) Wade Hampton Frost: an appreciation. *American Journal of Epidemiology*, 104: 392–395.

4 Sydenstricker E. (1925) The incidence of illness in a general population group; general results of a morbidity survey from December 1, 1921 through March 31, 1924 in Hagerstown, Md. *Public Health Reports*, 40: 279–291.

5 Sydenstricker E. (1926) A study of illness in a general population group. *Public Health Reports*, 39: Report No. 61.

6 Frost WH. (1933) Risk of persons in familial contact with pulmonary tuberculosis. *American Journal of Public Health*, 23: 426–432.

7 Frost WH. (1938) The familial aggregation of infectious disease. *American Journal of Public Health*, 28: 7–13.

8 Frost WH. (1939) The age selection of mortality from tuberculosis in successive decades. *American Journal of Hygiene*, 30: 91–96.

9 Frost WH. (1928) Infection, immunity and disease in the epidemiology of diphtheria, with special reference to some studies in Baltimore. *Journal of Preventive Medicine*, 2: 325–343.

10 Pearl R. (1924) Alcohol and Life Duration. *British Medical Journal*, 1: 948–950.

11 Rammelkamp CH, Denny FW, Wannomaker LW. (1952) Studies on the epidemiology of rheumatic fever in the armed services. In: *Rheumatic Fever* Thomas C (ed). Minneapolis, MN: University of Minnesota.

12 Stebbins EL, Ingraham HS, Read EA. (1937) Milk borne streptococcic infection. *American Journal of Public Health*, 27: 1259–1266.

13 Maxcy KF. (1926) An epidemiologic study of endemic typhus (Brill's disease) in the South-Eastern United States, with special reference to its mode of transmission. *Public Health Reports*, 41: 1.

14 Thompson LP, Brundage DK, Russell AE, Bloomfield JJ. (1928) The health of workers in dusty trades. The health of workers in a Portland cement plant. *Public Health Bulletin*, Report No.176 (April).

15 Goldberger J, Wheeler GA, Sydenstricker E. (1920) A study of the relation of diet to pellagra incidence in several textile communities of South Carolina in 1916. *Public Health Reports*, 35: 648–713.

16 Warren BS, Sydenstricker E. (1918) The relation of wages to Public Health. *American Journal of Public Health*, 8: 883–887.

17 Winslow CEA. (1923) *The Evolution and Significance of the Modern Public Health Campaign*. New Haven, CT: Yale University Press.

18 Amberson JB, McMahon BT, Pinner M. (1931) A clinical trial of sanocrysin in pulmonary tuberculosis. *Annual Review Tuberculosis*, 24: 401–425.

19 Wells CW, Flaherty EW, Smith HH. (1944) Results obtained in man with the use of a vaccine of heat killed tubercle bacilli. *American Journal of Hygiene*, 41: 116–121.

20 Trendley Dean H. (1938) Endemic fluorosis and its relation to dental caries. *Public Health Reports*, 53: 1443–1452.

21 Dean HT, Trendley A, Francis A, Elvolve E. (1942) Domestic water and dental caries. *Public Health Reports*, 57: 1155–1179.

22 McKay FS. (1942) Mass control of dental caries. *American Journal of Public Health*, 38: 828–832.

23 Klein H, Palmer CE, Knutson JW. (1938) Studies on dental caries. I: Dental status and dental needs of elementary school children. *Public Health Reports*, 53: 751–765.

24 Pearl R. (1938) Tobacco smoking and longevity. *Science*, 87: 216–217.

25 Pearl R. (1929) Cancer and tuberculosis. *American Journal of Hygiene*, 9: 97–159.

26 Berkson J. (1955) The statistical study of association between smoking and lung cancer. *Proceedings of the Mayo Clinic*, 30: 319–348.

27 Gilliam AG. (1961) personal communication.

28 Committee on the costs of medical care. (1932) American Medical Association. *Medical Care for the American People (final report)*. Chicago: University of Chicago Press.

29 Falk IS. (1974) In: *The Challenge of Facts. Selected Public Health Papers of E Sydenstricker*. Kasius RV, Prodist, NY (Eds). Health Policy: Commentary, 95–107.

30 Zinsser H. (1935) *Rats, Lice and History*. Boston, MA: Little, Brown and Co.

31 Webster LT. (1946) Experimental Epidemiology. Part I: Phenomena of epidemiology. *Medicine*, 25: 77–109.

32 Fee E. (1932) *Disease and Discovery. A history of the Johns Hopkins School of Hygiene and Public Health*. Baltimore, MD: Johns Hopkins University Press.

33 Paul JR. (1938) *Clinical Epidemiology*, 17: 539–541.

3. Epidemiological Public Health Research 1945–1998

The United Kingdom with comparison to the United States

This chapter covers EPHR in the years from 1945 to 1998, first for the United Kingdom and then for the United States. As with chapter 2, references for the two parts are carried at the end of each.

THE UNITED KINGDOM

Both the amount and the quality of EPHR carried out in this period in the UK were of a completely different magnitude to the first period. To try to determine the most important work, a group of senior academics was convened (see Note on p.69) and we discussed what had been achieved. The individuals chosen represented various areas of epidemiological and public health research interests, ages and locations within the United Kingdom to obtain a wide-ranging picture. Consensus on the most significant research during the period was reached with remarkable ease and the subsequent discussion reflects both the diversity of the work and the group's assessment of the most productive areas of study. Reference is made to representative publications and is not intended to be exhaustive.

Infectious / Communicable Disease

This group of conditions receded as major causes of mortality and serious morbidity and so attracted diminishing EPHR attention. Techniques for investigation and control of outbreaks of infectious disease had improved. It is not the intention here to elaborate on all the many good investigations of individual outbreaks – for example, of legionella, typhoid, or streptococcus. It is worth, however, noting some of the major methodological advances that were made, as well as to substantive new work on populations which led to better understanding of mechanisms of spread and methods of control.

Techniques

Major laboratory advances were made in mechanisms of characterising infecting organisms – for example, by phage-typing of staphylococci (REO Williams and P Jeavons) and enteric pathogens (ES Anderson) and by serotyping salmonellas (Joan Taylor) so that it became easier to identify causative agents and their routes of spread and to direct specific control measures.[1-3]

Methods of investigation of air hygiene were developed, in particular by Williams and Lidwell,[4] which led to a far better understanding of how airborne bacterial particles were spread and to better control of nosocomial infections in hospitals.

Development and dissemination of standardised reagents and laboratory procedures and the introduction of methods of quality control through the use of duplicate measurement, reference specimens and reagents were applied in most biochemical, microbiological and haematological laboratories.[5,6] This enabled epidemiologists, as well as clinicians, to have far more reliable tools available both in EPHR studies and in clinical practice. The current methods of molecular epidemiology have developed through the use of biomarkers of varying complexity.

Developments in microbiological classification procedures[7] have also greatly improved the precision with which different species and sub-types can be identified and thus the detail in which EPHR studies of their respective roles can be carried out.

Acute Respiratory Disease and Family Studies

Sir James Spence, Professor of Child Health in Newcastle, pioneered the investigation and follow-up of a group of 1000 families in Newcastle from the birth of an index child. The description of life and illness in the first year of life of this group[8] provided an illuminating account of how acute illnesses, particularly respiratory, occurred and spread in families, and the influence of factors such as family size, school terms, housing. The families were carefully followed and their illness experience recorded. These results have provided an important description of the development of health and disease in the early years of life.[9,10]

The technique of following up large birth cohorts was also used by Douglas on the early years of life[11] and others in 1947, 1958 and subsequently.[12-14] These latter studies were not directed solely at infectious disease but focused also on educational, social and environmental factors and their effect on the health and development of children and adults over time. Similar studies, directed by Dingle, were taking place in Cleveland.[15]

The problems of infectious disease – particularly acute respiratory disease – were also tackled in a group of families around St Mary's Hospital, London.[16] Studies in closed communities in the Royal Air Force led to a much better understanding of the role of different agents in the aetiology of these conditions.[17,18] Hope Simpson, a general practitioner, supported by the MRC and Public Health Laboratory Service (PHLS), undertook studies in a general practice in Cirencester equipped with a microbiological laboratory, so that all cases occurring in a general practice could be investigated immediately.[19,20] There were several pandemics of influenza which, in 1957 and 1968 in particular, led to detailed viral epidemiological studies that have provided us with a great deal of knowledge on how the virus spreads, its relation to population immunity and how outbreaks evolve in the community.[21,22]

Vaccine Developments

Major developments occurred with the design and execution of a large study of BCG vaccine in school children. This established both the safety and the efficacy of this vaccine, which had been under a cloud since the episode in Lübeck, Germany when a faulty batch of BCG containing live tubercle bacilli led to the deaths of 72 children.[23] Various other vaccines have been developed over the past 50 years – for example, pertussis, polio, measles, rubella, and HIB. One of the characteristics of EPHR research has been the development of careful, meticulous large trials of safety and efficacy for these new agents; specific examples of this include pertussis, rubella and measles.[24-31] This has enabled a better, safer and easier regime for immunisation to be administered to children so that in recent years the coverage of the eligible groups has been 90% or greater.

Questions also arose in this period about the effectiveness as well as the side-effects of pertussis vaccine. Careful investigations were carried out to enable estimates to be made on the likelihood of encephalitic events after vaccination, and more purified, even safer, vaccines were developed.[23-25]

Infectious Disease Surveillance

The concern with the safety of vaccines, and the possibilities of control and intervention of communicable diseases, led to the introduction of interesting, novel methods of routine surveillance.[29,30,31] These could reliably both detect the occurrence of new conditions and monitor the appearance of the "old ones", such as influenza, and took three main forms.

First came the routine reporting and publication in the Communicable Disease Report of the number and types of isolations in a number of laboratories linked to a central coordinating centre.[32]

Secondly, the Royal College of General Practitioners Research Unit coordinated a number of practices throughout the United Kingdom which routinely recorded and reported on the number and type of consultation.[33,34] This national scheme has been valuable not only in the recognition of the occurrence and importance of infectious disease but has also been instrumental in the surveillance of other conditions, such as the side effects of the "pill" discussed later in this chapter.[35] The development of this can be related to the earlier work by Pickles on disease in a general practice. [36]

Thirdly, new methods of surveillance have helped in the identification of new and emerging infections such as HIV, new variant Creutzfeldt Jakob Disease (vCJD), drug-resistant TB, and sexually transmitted diseases (STDs)[37,38] and in some of these enabled appropriate, effective control measures to be taken. In some instances, for example, legionnaires' disease, the presence of a good surveillance system has also improved the possibilities of treatment through early recognition and intervention.

Surveillance methods have, of course, been greatly improved by the development of computing and rapid means of communication (for example, the CDSC e-network) so that now rapid electronic means are available to alert appropriate agencies, including local communicable disease practitioners and laboratories, to any dangerous outbreak or recognition of a new agent.

The development of computing and computing power has also enabled much progress in the construction of mathematical models of the transmission and control of infectious disease. These have been used to evaluate different immunisation strategies – for example, for measles and rubella – and the prediction of epidemic evolution – for example, HIV/AIDS and vCJD.[39]

Methodology

Perhaps the most important contributions of EPHR between 1945 and 1970 in the UK have been in the development of various methods and techniques which can be used for both the investigation and the solution of clinical and public health problems. It is difficult to single out the most important contributions but they can usefully be classified under the following headings.

Questionnaires

For the investigation of various problems and conditions in populations, it is necessary to have available methods of questioning individuals as well as accurately measuring specific characteristics such as blood pressure, lung function and biochemical values.

Although this method of enquiry had been used for many years, in particular for social enquiries, its development for obtaining valid data on medical symptoms was a novelty. One of the best and earliest examples was the Medical Research Council Questionnaire on Respiratory Symptoms developed by Fletcher and colleagues.[40,41] The questionnaire was developed between about 1956 and 1960. It was translated into many languages and used in several hundred studies of chronic bronchitis in different parts of the world. It has served as a model for a number of respiratory disease questionnaires developed by other groups such as the American Thoracic Society, the International Union Against Tuberculosis and Lung Disease, and the National Coal Board.

Its development was important because the diagnosis of chronic bronchitis – or chronic respiratory disease as it has become known – depends almost entirely on the history an individual relates and not on pathognomonic physical signs or investigations. The use of standard instructions and training required for proper use of the questionnaire enabled estimates to be made of the frequency of the condition in both patients and populations defined in terms of standardised parameters, and allowed valid comparisons. Clinicians and investigators were thus able to discuss and measure a definite entity. The development of this questionnaire illustrated the need for careful attention to detail in population studies, since, for example, the phraseology used and the order of questions in the questionnaire could influence the answers given. If questions on smoking were asked before questions on cough or phlegm, for example, the frequency reported of the latter was less. It also enabled credible studies to be done to determine the prevalence and incidence of the condition in populations where the diagnosis of "chronic bronchitis" at the time was not recognised.[42,43] Other questionnaires on conditions such as angina followed rapidly.[44]

Methods of Measurement

The need for care in the measurement and interpretation of physical signs, investigations and so on began to be considered crucial at the end of the 1940s.

Yerushalmy[45] pioneered the need to be aware of the problem of interpretation and observer variability of chest X-rays. This became crucial in the diagnosis of pneumoconiosis where disability pensions and work ability were at stake.[46] Other examples rapidly accumulated, for example, in the interpretation of electrocardiograms (ECGs), and methods of coping with these problems were devised in the US as well as UK. [47,48]

The problem of blood pressure was particularly thorny. Two eminent Professors of Medicine, Platt[49] at Manchester and Pickering[50,51] at St Mary's, London and Oxford, held widely divergent views. The former considered that blood pressure was distributed in a bi-modal (or greater) way in a population, while the latter considered that it was distributed in a "normal" though skewed manner. This had important consequences both for the way in which patients were investigated and treated and for the "philosophy" of medicine.

If blood pressure was bi-modally distributed, then the condition was "controlled" largely genetically and individuals could be classified as normal or abnormal. If it was "normally" distributed, then the definition of abnormality was dependent on an operational criterion and the presence of more than one sign or symptom, which was determined by both genetic and environmental factors. Between 1958 and 1964 a number of investigations showed how fallible the standard method of blood pressure recording was[52,53] and various instruments were developed which enabled measurements to be made free of observer variability and technique. These findings showed that blood pressure was normally distributed skewed to the right with a long tail, and this has had consequences for policies and management of treatment of high blood pressure.

Similar methods were developed for the assessment of lung function.[54-56] These have had an important impact on the diagnosis and management of respiratory conditions such as asthma, chronic lung disease, and pneumoconiosis and on the conduct of epidemiological studies.

Population Studies

The need for EPHR studies to be carried out on defined population groups in order to obtain unbiased measures of the frequency of diseases and related variables had long been recognised. Application of this concept to populations in defined geographical areas was, however, slow to develop. Probably the most influential developments were made by Cochrane who studied defined population groups in the Rhondda and Vale of Glamorgan. He was instrumental in using these for a large variety of chronic disease problems, in addition to the investigation of pneumoconiosis in the Welsh valleys, the prime reason for their establishment. Other investigations – for example, on blood pressure – followed. Cochrane and his colleagues also developed the use of population groups for the investigation of the distribution of the values of specific characteristics such as length of metacarpals, haemoglobin, blood pressure and so on in normal populations in order to help in the use of these for diagnosis.[57-60]

Spence, a professor of paediatrics in Newcastle, used a somewhat similar methodology in his study of 1000 families in Newcastle to describe physical, social and environmental conditions and their relation to the incidence of illnesses as well as to other forms of development.

Longitudinal (Follow-up) Studies

Probably the most famous of all long-term follow-up studies was that of Hill and Doll of British Doctors to determine the relationship of smoking cigarettes to the development of lung cancer. The concept was simple – all doctors on the medical register received a note asking them about their smoking habits. More than two-thirds of the doctors replied. In order for a doctor to practise, presence on the medical register is mandatory. On the death of a doctor, the Registrar General automatically notifies the General Medical Council (GMC) (which maintains the medical register) so that the name is taken off the register. It was thus relatively easy, efficient, and cheap for Hill and Doll to ascertain the cause of death and its relationship to the previously reported smoking habit of the doctor. This study has been continued for more than 40 years – various modifications have been introduced over time in order to determine the effect, for example, of change in the smoking habit – and has probably been the most influential single study on the relationship of smoking to cancer of the lung and other diseases.[61–63]

The use of long-term follow-up studies was introduced first by Douglas[11] and then Butler[12,13] and others[64,65] for the investigation of a large variety of environmental, educational, physical, clinical and social factors on the development of disease, behavioural and other characteristics on all births in a defined month in 1947 and subsequently 1958. Both Douglas and Butler and their successors have been able to maintain contact with most of the original cohort by repeated mailing, visits and so on.[14]

More recently, investigations, such as those by Barker[66] and Davey Smith[67] have used the availability of records collected either at birth or, for example, at university medical entrance examinations in order to test a variety of hypotheses concerning risk factors for the development of disease or disease-related characteristics measured or ascertained in middle and old age. Although these have raised interesting hypotheses and findings, they have been subjected to criticism from various methodological perspectives.[68]

Evaluation of Screening Procedures
The development of mass X-rays for the identification of individuals with tuberculosis in the late 1940s greatly helped to advance the control of this disease. The concept of screening individuals for a variety of characteristics, such as blood pressure level and presence of cancer, is an extremely attractive one as it may enable effective treatment to be provided, thus preventing or at least mitigating the development of disease. Pressure from various sources to introduce screening tests in the UK increased in the early 1960s. The consequences of introducing such population measures for demands on resources rapidly became manifest. A good example of this was in cervical screening. The identification of abnormal cells from cervical screens was considered a precursor of cancer of the cervix. Once this finding was published, cervical screening became common – before either the resources to carry out universal cytology or evidence that this method of early diagnosis was effective in reducing the incidence of deaths from cancer of the cervix were available. Pathology laboratories were rapidly swamped by cytology requests.

The need for a proper policy on screening had been recognised by a medical officer in the Ministry of Health, Max Wilson.[69] As a result, a considered set of criteria was developed, and a number of others also became involved in the evaluation of screening procedures.[70,71] This has led to a much more effective and considered methodology in the evaluation of screening procedures so that there is now an agreed national policy of how to evaluate promising tests before they are recommended for widespread use. It has been shown that piecemeal introduction can not only lead to the wasteful use of scarce resources but can also lead to unnecessary anxiety and harm to individuals.[72]

Unbiased Statistical Methods
The development and application of randomised controlled trials by Bradford Hill in the treatment of tuberculosis with streptomycin was one of the greatest advances made in the evaluation of clinical treatment.[73]

It has since been developed and applied to a large number of procedures and evaluations of public health measures, such as vaccines. Although such trials are not an exclusively EPHR domain, they were nonetheless largely developed by epidemiologists and have led to enormous advances both in our knowledge of the causes of diseases and also in our ability to assess the effectiveness of interventions.

Other statistical methods,[74] particularly various forms of regression and logistic analysis, have enabled great advances to be made in the analysis of multiple risk factors and their relative importance in EPHR studies. This development of statistical methods has been linked to the parallel development of computers, which largely occurred first in the US.

Vital Statistics
The availability of national systems of registration of vital events such as birth, death and marriage, as well as accurate censuses, starting in the nineteenth century, enabled a wide variety of EPHR studies to be carried out – on changes in disease incidence in different social classes, for example,[75-77] and trends in mortality. Epidemiologists have become far more imaginative in the use of such readily available data since World War II.[78] This has been linked to the development of both hospital and general practitioner recording methods and regular household surveys of national samples that had been used during the war as barometers of opinions. The ability to trace individuals through the National

Health Service Register has enabled a large number of important studies to be done.[79,80] The development of record linkage in Scotland[81] enabled a number of studies to be done in that country,[82] based on the availability of good records from birth to death. Although a similar method was also piloted in Oxford,[83] it has not yet been applied elsewhere in England. The longitudinal survey introduced by the National Office of Vital Statistics has also been an important advance.[84]

The use of national household surveys[85,86] has been extended in recent times. After the appearance of HIV/AIDS, for example, the method was used to determine the pattern of sexual behaviour in national population samples in the UK,[87] thus going much further than some of the limited sample or "laboratory" studies by Masters and others in the USA. The use of such a survey to investigate sexual practices was, as one might expect, extremely controversial, but after the use of public funds for the purpose was vetoed, it was supported, eventually, by the Wellcome Trust. The results have helped in the formulation of appropriate prevention strategies and health education.

Major Disease / Risk Factor Studies

The application of epidemiological methods to the investigations of chronic disease burgeoned rapidly after the end of World War II.

Probably the greatest stimulus to these were the studies of Doll and Hill[61–63,88] on cancer of the lung and cigarette smoking. Starting with a model case-control study, followed by an efficient and effective longitudinal study, this developed methodology, tackled an important problem and produced highly relevant results which rapidly began to influence health policy – and perhaps most importantly, established the acceptability of epidemiology as an important tool in the investigation of chronic disease. It is not my intention here to describe these well-known studies which have been extensively covered by others.

Air Pollution – Lung Health

The 1952 London smog episode, which was associated with about 3000 excess deaths in London over a three-week period, was the stimulus for a large number of studies that increased knowledge of causation, leading to efforts to clean up the environment and to significant improvements in health. The smog episode in early December 1952 was particularly intense. The lack of concern for its consequences for human health was exemplified by the newspaper headlines of prize cattle dying at the Smithfield Show which was taking place at this time. The realisation that there was a major human catastrophe was first reported by florists who were unable to meet the demand for flowers at funerals.[89]

This episode resulted in a huge expansion of research into chronic respiratory disease. The studies of Lawther and Waller were directed particularly at the acute effects of pollution.[90,91] Several studies of mortality statistics, such as those by Pemberton,[92] described the geographical, secular, and demographic distribution of the disease. Fletcher, as described above, initiated the development of field methods for study of chronic respiratory conditions. Reid,[93] in a particularly imaginative series of studies on postal workers working indoors and outdoors, was able to describe the importance of the outdoor environment, and presumably air pollution independently of tobacco smoking habits, in the causation of chronic effects. This was taken further in both national and international studies [94] in which the relative contributions of smoking and outdoor air pollution to the prevalence of respiratory symptoms and disease were disentangled. Fletcher,[95] in a prospective study of London Transport bus and underground train repair and maintenance workers and Post Office Savings Bank office workers, was able to identify the prognostic significance of symptoms and lung function in the development of chronic respiratory diseases.

These various studies, as well as simultaneous investigations in occupational groups exposed to dusty environments, such as coal miners and pottery workers, were able to influence the development of appropriate control strategies and clearly demonstrated the overwhelming importance of cigarette smoking in the causation of chronic respiratory disease.[96]

Coronary Heart Disease (CHD)
During this period CHD rapidly attained a prominent place as a major cause of death and disability in the Western world. There was evidence from the analysis of the records of pathological specimens retained, particularly at the London Hospital,[97] that the increase was a real one, and was not the result solely of changes in terminology or diagnostic habits.

In the United States a series of longitudinal studies was started by Dawber and his colleagues in Framingham, Mass. In the United Kingdom, Jerry Morris at the Medical Research Council Social Medicine Research Unit started a series of extremely imaginative studies. Perhaps the most significant of these was his study of bus drivers and conductors.[98] This showed that, although the incidence of angina and myocardial infarction was not very different between the two groups, the case fatality was greater in bus drivers. This finding was surprising since in the 1950s and early 1960s the conductors were thought to be most exposed to stress. They were, however, far more active than the drivers, going up and down stairs in the double-deckers. These conclusions had to be interpreted with some caution – Morris was able to obtain from London Transport records of the uniform sizes of the individuals on entry to either driving or conducting in London Transport. The bus drivers tended to require larger uniforms than the conductors, particularly as measured by the waist of the trousers – that is, they were different in physique (and perhaps other characteristics) on entry into employment and it may be that the larger men chose to be drivers. Other studies by Morris and Paffenbarger in the United States, however, demonstrated the important preventive effect of exercise on the development of coronary heart diseases.

Rose was another eminent worker in this field, particularly in the development of standardised tools that could be used for the investigation of CHD. He and Reid began the studies of heart disease in civil servants which, some 20 years later, have enabled interesting findings to be made on the incidence of CHD in relation to a variety of social and psychological factors, illuminating the problem of inequalities in health in individuals in similar employment but at different levels in the hierarchy.[99–101]

Asthma

As with other respiratory diseases, some valuable studies were carried out on asthma, another chronic disease increasing in frequency. Perhaps one of the most interesting was an "outbreak" of acute deaths of asthma in the late 1960s observed by Doll and Speizer.[102,103] This was linked to the introduction of Beta-blockers which exacerbated the disease – and has led to major changes in their formulation. More recently Burney, Anderson and others have made major advances in our understanding of the relationship of asthma to allergy and other environmental agents.[104–107]

Medical Radiation and Leukaemia

Exposure to radiation as a health hazard was best illustrated by the explosion of the atomic bomb. The health hazards of X-rays were well known from effects such as burns and studies on mortality rates of radiologists (carried out in the US). The realisation that diagnostic radiation could do harm, however, was first demonstrated by Alice Stewart.[108] She showed that the children of mothers who received a diagnostic abdominal X-ray during pregnancy were at risk of developing leukaemia in the first five years of life. These findings were, at first, strongly challenged by Doll, but later also confirmed by him and others.[109]

The hazards of X-rays and their association with leukaemia were also shown by Court Brown and Doll in a series of studies of adults treated by radiotherapy for Ankylosing Spondylitis.[110] These investigations have led to a complete change in practice in the investigation of pregnant mothers and the treatment of various conditions, as well as the introduction of standards for exposure to diagnostic and therapeutic irradiation.

More recently, Draper,[111,112] Gardner,[113–115] Heasman[116] and others have been active in the investigation of the health hazards of exposure to atomic energy irradiation as a result of employment in industrial plants and accidental release of contaminated products.

Aspirin and CHD

The role of aspirin both in the prevention of CHD and in the initial treatment of a myocardial infarct and of stroke was highlighted and discovered by Elwood.[117] It has led to a dramatic effect on CHD mortality and morbidity.

The Contraceptive Pill – Thrombosis and Embolism in Women

Vessey and Kay,[35,118] among others, have investigated the occurrence of venous thrombosis and embolism in women taking the pill as a preventative agent. Their work has led to a series of modifications of these highly desirable agents so that the risk in women on this medication is now much lower.

Blood Pressure

As referred to earlier, it was Pickering who first suggested that the distribution of blood pressure in a population was "normally" distributed.[50,51] Miall carried out a study of blood pressure in a normal population in South Wales and was able to confirm Pickering's hypothesis and to describe the distribution of blood pressure in the two genders and the variation with age.[59,60] This has been of great importance in the development of our knowledge of who should be treated and when.

Congenital Malformations

Lowe,[119] Leck[120] and others contributed much to our knowledge of the frequency of a variety of congenital malformations and their possible environmental and genetic determinants. This has been of particular benefit in the identification of new hazards, such as thalidomide, and the introduction of appropriate, feasible methods of surveillance and control.

Dental Disease

It is difficult to identify any specific enquiries in the UK associated with the enormous improvements that have occurred in dental health in the past 50 years – but the meticulously repeated surveys of caries in school children have documented the advances made as a result of improvements in social and environmental conditions.[121]

Psychiatry

The role of epidemiology and public health in advances in the prevention, treatment and care of psychiatric conditions is often neglected. This is due in part to the inherent difficulties of diagnosis, terminology and societal norms in the study of behavioural illnesses. The studies of Tooth and Brooke[79] and others were, however, largely instrumental in the change from institutional to community care in psychiatry. Kushlick,[122] John and Lorna Wing[123-125] and others [126,127] in their very careful studies of both institutions and populations have been instrumental in the change in methods of care and treatment of the mentally ill and handicapped. Rutter, in his studies on the Isle of Wight, has been able to provide a description of the development of different behaviours in children and adolescents.[128]

Carstairs[129] contributed to our knowledge of the effect of a variety of social factors on mental health. Shepherd,[130] Goldberg[131] and others were particularly responsible for the development of epidemiological tools in psychiatry and the ability to measure these conditions reliably in populations. It is often forgotten that the major preventative measure for reducing the burden of psychiatric deaths and illnesses was the introduction of measles and mumps vaccines which prevented the occurrence of measles and mumps encephalitides. The seminal work of Reid[132,133] on bomber pilot "fatigue" should not be forgotten, in view of current concerns with post-traumatic stress disorders in servicemen.

Nutrition

As we have recorded previously,[134] the nutrition of people in the UK changed greatly as a result of the introduction of rationing in 1939. After the war, undernutrition was no longer a problem, so that research and education in this field became neglected. Although there were occasional concerns at the reappearance of rickets in isolated population groups – in deprived children in Glasgow, for example, and in Indian children fed on a diet deficient in Vitamin D – there were no major EPHR studies in this area.

The election of a Conservative government in 1970, however, led to major changes in food policy.[135] Among these were measures to restrict the issue of free milk to pregnant mothers, free milk to children age below 5 years, and free milk to school children aged over 7 years. It is of particular interest that the policy-makers, politicians and civil servants were persuaded to mount a series of large-scale observational and experimental studies to determine whether these changes in food policy had any harmful effects in either the short or the long term.[136] Some of these systems of surveillance were continued for 20 years and provide an excellent record of secular changes in height and weight in primary school children – and in particular the increase in obesity in these children, particularly girls.

The other major nutritional studies were concerned with the association of the protective effect of fibre on colon cancer and heart disease, following the observations of Burkitt and Hutt in Uganda.[137,138]

Occupational health

Although it had long been recognised that some industries posed particular health hazards, their precise nature and means of prevention were elucidated only in the 1960s and 1970s. Arguably, the most notable of these epidemiological studies were those by Schilling[139] on the nature and cause of byssinosis in cotton workers. Pneumoconiosis in coal workers was similarly tackled in some exemplary studies by Cochrane,[140] Gilson,[141] Rogan[142] and others. Advances in these areas were largely the result of the ability to make reliable quantitative measures of harm done through exposure to a hazard by the use of appropriate questionnaires, X-ray examinations and ventilatory function measurements discussed above.

Remarkable observational studies linked to appropriately developed methods of statistical enquiry enabled Case[143] to specify the risks of development of bladder cancer in rubber workers and Newhouse[144] mesothelioma in individuals exposed to asbestos fibres. These methods were also applied to the investigation of occupational TB and occupational fatalities and trauma. These industries are now far safer because appropriate legislation has been introduced to control and mitigate the hazards.

Philosophy of Medicine

With advances in methods of treatment and possibilities for investigation and prevention, some workers began to question the advances and effects medicine had made in improving health. Most noteworthy here was McKeown who, in a scholarly monograph,[145] examined the trends in mortality over time and attempted to assess the contributions medicine might have made to these. His conclusions were that although medical science had made a contribution, especially since the introduction of antibiotics and chemotherapeutic agents, the effect was relatively very small compared to the effect of changes in nutrition, in particular, associated with increases in wealth. These observations raised a great deal of controversy, particularly as they were published at about the same time as those by some sociologists. Illich,[146] in particular, questioned the role and powers of medicine generally. The most cogent criticism was, however, by Szreter,[147] who suggested that McKeown had not given sufficient credit to changes in hygiene, which he considered to have played an important role.

Health Services Research

With the advent of the National Health Service a number of studies began to determine whether it was achieving its goals. Logan's studies showing the marked differences between Manchester and Liverpool in the availability of hospital facilities and the differences in uptake drew attention to the large inequalities that existed between different areas but also to the fact that gains in efficiency could be made.[148] The concept that we knew little about the effectiveness of health services was highlighted by Cochrane in his Rock Carling monograph.[149] This was, without doubt, the major stimulus to the development of a large number of studies in a variety of locations. The Nuffield Provincial Hospital Trust publications, Portfolio for Health 1 and 2,[150,151] describe the developments and range of studies being carried out. Of particular note was the development and application of the Randomised Controlled Trial (RCT) in health services research. One prime example of this application was the demonstration of the lack of benefit of intensive hospital care in the management of acute myocardial infarction compared with home care at a time when modern methods of treatment with thrombolytics were not available.[152] A second example was an RCT of multiphasic screening in general practice which showed that screening did not produce any benefit compared to routine care but, if introduced, would increase NHS costs by about 10%.[153]

The need to be concerned about the use of health services resources was perhaps best illustrated by the acceptance that, before any new screening procedure was introduced into practice, certain criteria of efficiency and effectiveness needed to be met. At this time also a series of studies on the variation in length of hospital stay and types of investigation[154,155] highlighted the wide variations which existed in clinical practice in the United Kingdom. These led to further studies on, for example, the lack of harm caused by discharging patients early after minor operations,[156] which have provided evidence on how clinical practice could and should be changed. This has now been followed by the formalisation of health services research in the creation of a Directorate of Research and Development within the health service structure.[157]

But before this there had already been major changes in health care in the UK – perhaps the most important of these was the introduction of community-based mental health care, referred to above.

The UK also pioneered the application of "avoidable mortality" in assessing the quality of health care and highlighting areas where change was required.[158] This heralded a greater concern with the outcome of clinical services. Now the NHS has developed a much greater concern with not only the processes of care, but also their outcomes and the application and use of evidence in the consideration of appropriate methods of treatment.

This was a period when EPHR came of age in the UK and began to catch up with and at times overtake in quantity and quality, research being carried out across the Atlantic.

REFERENCES

1 Wilson GS, Miles AA. (1955) *Topley and Wilson's Principles of Bacteriology and immunity.* London: Edward Arnold.

2 Williams REO, Rippon JE. (1952) Bacteriophage typing of staph areus *Journal of Hygiene, Cambridge*, 50: 320–353.

3 Blair JE, Williams REO. (1961) Phage typing of staphlylococci. *Bulletin of the World Health Organization*, 24: 771–784.

4 Lidwell OM, Williams REO. (1954) *British Medical Journal* , 2: 959–961.

5 Whitehead TP, Morris LO. (1969) Methods of quality control. *Annals of Clinical Biochemistry*, 6: 94.

6 Whitehead TP. (1973) The Wolfson Laboratories. In: *Portfolio for Health 2.* Oxford: Oxford University Press for the Nuffield Provincial Hospitals Trust.

7 Cowan ST. (1965) Principles and practice of bacterial taxonomy – a forward look. *Journal of General Microbiology*, 39: 143.

8 Spence J, Walton WS, Miller FJW, Court SDM. (1954) *A Thousand Families in Newcastle upon Tyne.* London: Oxford University Press.

9 Miller FJW, Court SDM, Walton WS, Knox EG. (1960) *Growing up in Newcastle upon Tyne.* London: Oxford University Press.

10 Miller FJW, Court SDM, Knox EG, Brandon S. (1974) *The School Years in Newcastle upon Tyne.* London: Oxford University Press.

11 Douglas JWB, Blomfield JM. (1958) *Children Under Five.* London: George Allen and Unwin.

12 Butler NR. (1961) Perinatal Mortality Survey under the auspices of the National Birthday Trust. *Proceedings of the Royal Society Medicine*, 54: 1089–1092.

13 Butler NR. (1961) National survey of perinatal mortality first results. *British Medical Journal*, 1: 1313–1315.

14 Goldstein H. (1983) A study of response rates of 16 year olds in the National Child Development Study. In: *Growing up in Great Britain*. Fogelman K (ed). London: Macmillan.

15 Dingle JH, Badger GF, Jordan WS. (1964) *Illness in the Home. A Study of 25,000 Illnesses in a Group of Cleveland Families*. Cleveland, OH: The Press of Western Reserve University.

16 Cruickshank R. (1958) A survey of respiratory illnesses in a sample of families in London. In: *Recent Studies in Epidemiology*. Pemberton J, Willard H (eds). Oxford: Blackwell. pp 67–79.

17 McDonald JC, Wilson JS, Thorburn WB, et al. (1958) Acute respiratory disease in the RAF 1955–7. *British Medical Journal*, 2: 721–724.

18 McDonald JC, Miller DL, Zuckerman AJ, Pereira M, et al. (1962) Coe (coxsackie A21) virus, parainfluenza virus and other respiratory virus infections in the RAF 1958–1960. *Journal Hygiene Cambridge*, 60: 235–248.

19 Miller DL, Hope Simpson RE, Court D. (1973) Collaborative studies of ARI in GP, and children in hospital. *Symposium Postgrad. Medical Journal*, 49: 749 et. Seq.

20 Medical Research Council Committee on ARI. (1965) Collaborative study of aetiology of ARI in Britain 1961–1964. *British Medical Journal*, 2: 319–326.

21 Stuart Harris CH. (1953) *Influenza and Other Virus Infections of the Respiratory Tract*. London: Edward Arnold.

22 Miller DL, Pereira M, Clarke M, et al. (1971) Epidemiology of HK influenza/68. *British Medical Journal*, 1: 475.

23 Sutherland I, Springett VH. (1989) The effects of the scheme for BCG vaccination of school children in England and Wales and the consequences of discontinuing the scheme at various dates. *Journal of Epidemiological and Community Health*, 43: 15–24.

24 Medical Research Council. (1959) Vaccination against whooping cough. Final Report. *British Medical Journal*, 1: 994–1000.

25 Dudgeon JA, Marshall WC, Peckham CS. (1969) Rubella vaccine trials in adults and children. Comparison of three attenuated vaccines. *American Journal of Diseases in Children*,118: 237–243.

26 Dudgeon JA, Marshall WC, Peckham CS, et al. (1971) Immunisation against rubella. A study to determine the place of rubella vaccination as a selective procedure in a comprehensive immunisation programme. *Practitioner*, 207: 782–790.

27 Medical Research Council. (1966) Measles Vaccine Committee of the MRC. *British Medical Journal*, 1: 441.

28 Miller C. (1987) Live measles vaccine: a 21 year follow up. *British Medical Journal*, 295: 22–24.

29 Miller DL, Ross EM, Alderslade R, et al. (1981) Pertussis immunisation and serious neurological illness in children. *British Medical Journal*, 282: 1595–1599.

30 Miller DL, Madge N, Diamond J, et al. (1993) Pertussis immunisation and serious acute neurological illness in children. *British Medical Journal*, 307: 1171–1176.

31 Miller E. (1999) Overview of recent clinical trials of acellular pertussis vaccines. *Biologicals*, 27: 79–86.

32 Galbraith NS. (1989) CDSC: from Cox to Acheson. *Community Medicine*, 11: 187–199.

33 Fleming DM, Norbury CA, Crombie DL. (1991) Annual and seasonal variation in the incidence of common diseases. Occasional paper. *Royal College of General Practitioners*, 53: 1–24.

34 Crombie DL, Fleming DM. (1988) Practice activity analysis. Occasional paper. *Royal College of General Practitioners*,41: 1–47.

35 Kay CR. The Royal College of General Practitioners contraceptive study. (1975) *A longitudinal controlled survey of effects of oral contraception on health.* Manchester University PhD.

36 Pemberton J. (1972) *Will Pickles of Wensleydale.* London: Royal College of General Practitioners.

37 Tillett HE, Galbraith NS, Overton SE, Porter K. (1988) Routine surveillance data on AIDS and HIV infections in the UK: a description of the data available and their use for short-term planning. *Epidemiology and Infection*, 100: 152–169.

38 Galbraith NS, Young SE, Pusey JJ, et al. (1984) Mumps surveillance in England and Wales 1962–81. *Lancet*, 1: 91–94.

39 Anderson RM, Nokes DJ. (1997) Mathematical models of transmission and control. In: *Oxford Textbook of Public Health.* 3rd edition. Detels R, Holland W, McEwen J, Omenn GS (Eds). Vol. II. Oxford:Oxford University Press.

40 Medical Research Council's Committee on the Aetiology of Chronic Bronchitis. (1960) Standardised questionnaire on respiratory symptom. *British Medical Journal*, 2: 1665.

41 Fletcher CM. (1958) Difficulties of Definition and Observer Error. In: *Recent Studies in Epidemiology.* Pemberton J, Willard H (Eds). Oxford: Blackwell Scientific Publications, pp 37–42.

42 Meneely GR, Paul O, Dorn HF, Harrison TR. (1960) Cardiopulmonary semantics. *JAMA*, 174: 1628–1629.

43 Reid DD. (1960) Cardiorespiratory Disease as a field for international research. *American Journal of Public Health*, 50: Part II, 53–59.

44 Rose GA. (1964) Chest Pain Questionnaire. In: *Comparability in International Epidemiology.* Acheson RM (Ed). New York: Milbank Memorial Fund, pp 32–39.

45 Yerushalmy J, Garland LH, Harkness JT, Hinshaw HC, et al. (1951) Tuberculosis. *American Review of Tuberculosis*, 64: 225–248.

46 Gilson JC, Hugh-Jones P. (1955) *Lung function in Coalworkers Pneumoconiniosis*. London: Medical Research Council Special Report Series.

47 Higgins ITT. (1964) Ischaemic Heart Disease: the problem. In: *Comparability in International Epidemiology*. Acheson RM (Ed). New York: Milbank Memorial Fund, pp 23–31.

48 Blackburn HA, Keys A, Simonsene E, Rautaharju P, et al. (1960) The Electrocardiogram in Population Studies:a Classification System. *Circulation*, 21: 116–1175.

49 Platt R. (1959). The nature of essential hypertension. *Lancet*, 2: 55–57.

50 Pickering, GW. (1961).The nature of essential hypertension. In: *Epidemiology*. Pemberton J (Ed). London: Oxford University Press.

51 Pickering GW. (1963) The inheritance of arterial pressure. In: *Epidemiology*. Pemberton J (Ed). London: Oxford University Press, pp 97–114.

52 Holland WW. (1963) The reduction of observer variability in the measurement of blood pressure. In: *Epidemiology*. Pemberton J (Ed). London: Oxford University Press, pp 271–281.

53 Rose GA, Holland WW, Crowley EA. (1964) A Sphygmomanometer for Epidemiologists. *Lancet*, 1: 296–300.

54 Fletcher CM. (1963) Some problems of diagnostic standardization using clinical methods, with special reference to chronic bronchitis. In: *Epidemiology*. Pemberton J (Ed). London: Oxford University Press, pp 253–260.

55 McKerrow C. (1963) Standardization of respiratory function tests. In: *Epidemiology*. Pemberton J (Ed). London: Oxford University Press, pp 282–294.

56 Cochrane AL. (1963) Standardization of the radiological diagnosis of pneumoconiosis. In: *Epidemiology*. Pemberton J (Ed). London: Oxford University Press, pp 287–294.

57   Cochrane AL. (1965) Survey methods in a general population Rhondda Fach, S. Wales. In: *Comparability in International Epidemiology*. Acheson RM (Ed). New York: Milbank Memorial Fund, pp 326–332.

58   Elwood PC, Weddell JM. (1971) Epidemiology of some common conditions. *British Medical Bulletin*, 27: 32–36.

59   Miall WE, Oldham PD. (1955) Factors influencing arterial blood pressure in the general population. *Clinical Science*, 14: 459–488.

60   Miall WE, Oldham PD. (1958) A study of arterial blood pressure and its inheritance in a sample of the general population. *Clinical Science*, 17: 409–444.

61   Doll WR, Hill AB. (1954) The mortality of doctors in relation to their smoking habits. A preliminary report. *British Medical Journal*, 1: 1451–1455.

62   Doll WR, Hill, AB. (1956) Lung cancer and other causes of death in relation to smoking. *British Medical Journal*, 2: 1071–1081.

63   Doll R, Peto R, Wheatley K, et al. (1994) Mortality in relation to smoking: 40 years' observations on male British doctors. *British Medical Journal*, 309: 901–911.

64   Wadsworth MEJ, Kuh DJL. (1997) Childhood influences on adult health: a review of recent work from the British 1946 national birth cohort study, the MRC National Survey of Health Development. *Paediatrics and Perinatal Epidemiology*, 11: 2–20.

65   Power C. (1992) A review of child health in the 1958 birth cohort: National Child Development Study. *Paediatrics and Perinatal Epidemiology*, 6: 81–110.

66   Barker DJP (Ed). (1992) *Foetal and Infant Origins of Adult Disease*. London: British Medical Journal Publishing Group.

67   Davey Smith G, Kuh D. (1997) Does early nutrition affect later health: Views from the 1930s and 1980s. In: *The History of Nutrition in Britain in the 20th Century: Science, Scientists and Politics*. Smith D (Ed). London: Routledge.

68 Joseph KS, Kramer MS. (1996) Review of evidence on foetal and early childhood antecedents of adult chronic disease. *Epidemiologic Reviews*, 18: 158–174.

69 Wilson JMG, Jungner G. (1968) *Principles and practice of screening for disease.* Geneva: World Health Organisation.

70 Cochrane AL, Holland WW. (1971) Validation of screening procedures. *British Medical Bulletin*, 27(i): 3–8.

71 McKeown T. (1968) Validation of screening procedures. In: *Screening in Medical Care: Reviewing the Evidence.* Oxford: Oxford University Press for the Nuffield Provincial Hospitals Trust.

72 Holland WW, Stewart S. (1990) *Screening in Health Care: Benefit or Bane?* London: Nuffield Provincial Hospitals Trust.

73 British Medical Research Council. (1948) Streptomycin treatment of pulmonary tuberculosis. *British Medical Journal*, 2: 768–782.

74 Armitage P. (1971) *Statistical Methods in Medical Research.* Oxford: Blackwell Scientific Publications.

75 Heady JA, Heasman MA. (1959) *Social and Biological Factors in Infant Mortality.* London: HMSO.

76 Morris JN, Heady JA. (1955) Social and biological factors in infant mortality. Objects and methods. *Lancet*, 1: 343–349.

77 Morris JN, Heady JA. (1955) Mortality in relation to father's occupation. *Lancet*, 1: 554–559.

78 Benjamin B. (1959) *Elements of Vital Statistics.* London: George Allen & Unwin.

79 Tooth GC, Brooke EM. (1961) Trends in the mental health population. *Lancet*, 1: 710–713.

80 Watts SP, Acheson ED. (1967) Computer method for deriving hospital in-patient statistics based on the person as the unit. *British Medical Journal*, 4: 476–477.

81 Heasman MA, Clarke JA. (1979) Medical Record Linkage in Scotland. *Health Bulletin*, 37: 97–103.

82 Baldwin JA. (1971) Aspects of the epidemiology of mental illness: studies in record linkage. *International Psychiatry Clinics*, 8 (3): vii–xii.

83 Acheson ED. (1967) *Medical Record Linkage*. Nuffield Provincial Hospitals Trust. Oxford: Oxford University Press.

84 Fox AJ, Goldblatt PO. (1982) *Longitudinal Study: Socio-Economic Mortality differentials*. 1971–75. London: Office of Population Censuses and Surveys.

85 Stocks P. (1949) Sickness in the population of England and Wales, 1944–47. London: HMSO.

86 OPCS (Office of Population Censuses and Surveys). (1973) *General Household Survey: Introductory Report*. London: HMSO.

87 Johnson AM, Wadsworth J, Wellings K, Field J. (1994) *Sexual Attitudes and Life-Styles*. Oxford: Blackwell Scientific Publications.

88 Doll R, Hill AB. (1950) Smoking and carcinoma of the lung. A preliminary report. *British Medical Journal*, 2: 739–748.

89 Royal College of Physicians. (1970) *Air Pollution and Health*. London: Royal College of Physicians.

90 Lawther PJ. (1958) Climate, Air Pollution and Chronic Bronchitis. *Proceedings of the Royal Society of Medicine*, 51: 262–264.

91 Waller RE, Lawther PJ, Martin AE. (1969). *Clean Air and Health in London*. Proceedings of the Clean Air Conference, Eastbourne, 1969, Part I, 71–79. London: National Society for Clean Air.

92   Pemberton J, Goldberg C. (1954) Air pollution and bronchitis. *British Medical Journal*, 2: 567–570.

93   Fairbairn AS, Reid DD. (1958) Air pollution and other local factors in respiratory disease. *British Journal of Preventive and Social Medicine*, 12: 94–103.

94   Holland WW, Reid DD. (1965) The urban factor in chronic bronchitis. *Lancet*, 1: 445–448.

95   Fletcher CM, Peto R, Tinker C, Speizer FE. (1976) *The natural history of chronic bronchitis and emphysema. An eight year study of early chronic obstructive lung disease in working men in London.* Oxford: Oxford University Press.

96   Rogan JM, Attfield MD, Jacobsen M, et al. (1990) Role of dust in the working environment in development of chronic bronchitis in British coal miners. *British Journal of Industrial Medicine*, 30: 217–226.

97   Morris JN. (1951) Recent history of coronary heart disease. *Lancet*, 1: 69–73.

98   Morris JN, Kagan A, Pattison DC, Gardner MJ. (1966) Incidence and prediction of ischaemic heart disease in London busmen. *Lancet*, 2: 553–559.

99   Reid DD, Hamilton PJS, Keen H, et al. (1974) Cardiorespiratory disease and diabetes among middle-aged male civil servants: a study of screening and intervention. *Lancet*, 1: 469–473.

100   Reid DD, McCartney P, Jarrett RS, et al. (1976) Smoking and other risk factors for coronary heart disease in British Civil Servants. *Lancet*, 2: 979–983.

101   Rose G, Hamilton PJS, Keen H, et al. (1977) Myocardial ischaemia, risk factors and death from coronary heart disease. *Lancet*, 1:105–109.

102   Speizer FE, Doll R, Heaf P. (1968) Observations on the recent increase in mortality from asthma. *British Medical Journal*, 1: 335–339.

103   Speizer FE, Doll R, Heaf P, Strang LB. (1968) Investigation into use of drugs preceding deaths from asthma. *British Medical Journal*, 1: 339–343.

104   Anderson HR, Bailey P, West S. (1980) Trends in the hospital care of acute childhood asthma. *British Medical Journal*, 281: 1191–1194.

105   Anderson HR, Bland JM, Patel S, Peckham C. (1986) The natural history of asthma in childhood. *Journal of Epidemiology and Community Health*, 40: 121–129.

106   Burney PGJ. (1986) Asthma mortality in England and Wales: Evidence for a further increase. 1974–84. *Lancet*, 2: 323–326.

107   Burney PGJ, Britton JR, Chinn S, et al. (1987) Descriptive epidemiology of bronchial reactivity in an adult population: results from a community study. *Thorax*, 42: 38–44.

108   Stewart A. (1961) Aetiology of childhood leukaemia. *British Medical Journal*, 1: 452–460.

109   MacMahon B. (1962) Prenatal x-ray exposure and childhood cancer. *Journal of the National Cancer Institute*, 28: 1173–1191.

110   Court Brown WM, Doll R. (1957) *Leukaemia and Aplastic Anaemia in Patients Irradiated for Ankylosing Spondylitis*. London: HMSO.

111   Draper GJ, Little MP, Sorohan T, et al. (1997) Cancer in the offspring of radiation workers: a record linkage study. *British Medical Journal*, 315: 1181–1188.

112   Stiller CA, Draper GP. (1998) The epidemiology of cancer in children. In: *Cancer in Children*. Voute PA, Kalifa C, Barrett A (Eds). London: Oxford University Press, pp 1–20.

113   Gardner MJ, Snee MP, Hall A, et al. (1990) Results of case control study of leukaemia and lymphoma among young people near Sellafield nuclear plant in West Cumbria. *British Medical Journal*, 1: 423–429.

114   Gardner MJ, Hall AP, Snee MP, et al. (1990) Methods and basic data of case-control study of leukaemia and lymphoma among young people near Sellafield nuclear plant in West Cumbria. *British Medical Journal*, 1: 429–434.

115 Gardner MJ. (1991) Childhood cancer and nuclear installations. *Public Health*, 105: 277–285.

116 Heasman MA, Urquahart JD, Black RJ, et al. (1987) Leukaemia in young persons in Scotland. A study of its geographical distribution and relationships to nuclear installations. *Health Bulletin*, 45: 147–151.

117 Elwood PC, Cochrane AL, Brown ML, et al. (1974) A randomised controlled trial of acetylsalicylic acid in the secondary prevention of mortality from myocardial infarction. *British Medical Journal*, 1: 436–440.

118 Vessey MP, Doll R. (1968) Investigation of relation between use of oral contraceptives and thromboembolic disease. *British Medical Journal*, 2: 199–205.

119 Lowe CR. (1972) Congenital malformations and the problem of their control. *British Medical Journal*, 3: 515–520.

120 Leck I. (1976) Descriptive epidemiology of common malformations. *British Medical Bulletin*, 32: 45–52.

121 O'Brien M. (1994) *Children's Dental health in the UK*. London: HMSO.

122 Kushlick A. (1975) The need for residential care of the mentally handicapped. *British Journal of Psychiatry*, Special Number 9, 377–383.

123 Wing JK. (1962) Institutionalism in mental hospitals. *British Journal of Clinical Psychology*, 1: 38–51.

124 Wing JK. (1984) *Report of the Camberwell Psychiatric Register. 1964–1984*. London: MRC Social Psychiatry Unit, Institute of Psychiatry.

125 Wing L. (1981, 1982, 1983, 1984) *Evaluation of New Services to be Provided for Residents of Darenth Park Hospital*. London: MRC Social Psychiatry Unit Reports, Nos 1, 2, 3 and 4.

126 Grad J, Sainsbury P. (1966) Problems of caring for the mentally ill at home. *Proceedings of the Royal Society of Medicine*, 59: 20–23.

127   Sainsbury P, Grad J. (1966) Evaluating the community psychiatric service in Chichester. Aims and methods of research. *Milbank Memorial Fund Quarterly*, 44: 231–242.

128   Rutter M. (1979) *Changing Youth in a Changing Society*. Rock Carling Fellowship. London: Nuffield Provincial Hospitals Trust.

129   Carstairs GM. (1963) Standardisation of psychiatric judgements. In: *Epidemiology: Reports on Research and Teaching*. Pemberton J (Ed). London: Oxford University Press, pp 261–270.

130   Shepherd M, Cooper B, Brown AC, Kalton GW. (1981) *Psychiatric Illness in General Practice*. 2nd edition. London: Oxford University Press.

131   Goldberg DP, Cooper B, Eastwood MR, et al. (1970) A standardised psychiatric interview for use in community surveys. *British Journal of Preventive and Social Medicine*, 24: 18–23.

132   Reid DD. (1961) Precipitating proximal factors in the occurrence of mental disorders. Epidemiological evidence. *Milbank Memorial Fund Quarterly*, 39: 229–259.

133   Reid DD. (1948) Sickness and stress in operational flying. *British Journal of Social Medicine*, 2: 123–131.

134   Holland WW, Stewart S. (1998) *Public Health, the Vision and the Challenge*. London: Nuffield Trust.

135   Department of Health and Social Security. (1973) First report by the sub-committee on nutritional surveillance. *Reports on Health and Social Subjects*. No. 6. London: HMSO.

136   Rona RJ, Chinn S. (1999) *The National Study of Health and Growth*. London, Oxford: Oxford University Press.

137   Hutt MS, Burkitt D. (1965) Geographical distribution of cancer in East Africa: a new clinicopathological approach. *British Medical Journal*, 2: 719–722.

138   Hutt MS, Burkitt DP. (1973) Aetiology of Burkitt's Lymphoma. *Lancet*, 1: 439.

139   Mekky S, Roach SA, Schilling RS. (1967) Byssinosis among winders in the cotton industry. *British Journal of Industrial Medicine*, 2: 123–132.

140   Cochrane AL. (1973) Relation between radiographic categories of coalworkers' pneumoconiosis and expectation of life. *British Medical Journal*, 2: 532–534.

141   Gilson JC, Oldham PD. (1970) Coalworkers' pneumoconiosis. *British Medical Journal*, 4: 305.

142   Rogan J. (1970) Coalworkers' pneumoconiosis: a review. *Journal of Occupational Medicine*, 8: 321–324.

143   Case RA. (1966) Tumours of the urinary tract as an occupational disease in several industries. *Annals of the Royal College of Surgeons of England*, 39: 213–235.

144   Newhouse ML, Thompson H. (1965) Mesothelioma of pleura and peritoneum following exposure to asbestos in the London area. *British Journal of Industrial Medicine*, 22: 261–269.

145   McKeown T. (1976) *The Role of Medicine. Dream, Mirage or Nemesis*. Rock Carling Fellowship. London: Nuffield Provincial Hospitals Trust.

146   Illich I. (1995) *Limits of Medicine. Medical Nemesis. The Expropriation of Health*. London: Marion Boyars.

147   Szreter S. (1986) *The Importance of Social Intervention in Britain's Mortality Decline, c1850–1914, a Reinterpretation*. London: Centre for Economic Policy Research.

148   Logan RFL. (1972) *Dynamics of Medical Care: the Liverpool Study Into Use of Hospital Resources*. London: London School of Hygiene and Tropical Medicine.

149   Cochrane AL. (1973) *Effectiveness and Efficiency: Random Reflections on Health Services*. London: Nuffield Provincial Hospitals Trust.

150   McLachlan G (Ed). (1971) *Portfolio for Health 1*. London: Nuffield Provincial Hospitals Trust/Oxford University Press.

151   McLachlan G (Ed). (1971) *Portfolio for Health 2*. London: Nuffield Provincial Hospitals Trust/Oxford University Press.

152   Mather HG, Morgan DC, Pearson NG, et al. (1976) Myocardial infarction: a comparison between home and hospital care for patients. *British Medical Journal*, 1: 925–929.

153   SELSS. (1977) A controlled trial of multiphasic screening in middle-age: Results of the South-East London Screening study. *International Journal of Epidemiology*, 6: 357–363.

154   Heasman MA. (1964) How long in hospital? A study in variation in duration of stay for two common surgical conditions. *Lancet*, 2: 539–541.

155   Heasman MA, Carstairs V. (1971) In-patient management: variations in some aspects of practice in Scotland. *British Medical Journal*, 1: 495–498.

156   Waller J, Adler M, Creese A, Thorne S. (1978) *Early discharge from hospital for patients with hernia or varicose veins*. London: HMSO.

157   Peckham M. (1999) *A Model for Health*. Rock Carling Fellowship. London: Nuffield Trust.

158   Holland WW (Ed). (1988, 1991, 1993, 1997) *The European Community Atlas of "Avoidable mortality"*. Vol. I (1st edition), Vol. I (2nd edition), Vol. II (2nd edition), Vol. II (3rd edition). Oxford, London: Oxford University Press.

NOTE
Senior academic assessment group
Professor Peter Ellwood – MRC Epidemiological Research Unit, Cardiff.
Professor C du V Florey – University of Dundee.
Professor G Knox – University of Birmingham.
Professor DL Miller – St Mary's Hospital Medical School (now Imperial College) University of London.
Professor J Pemberton – University of Sheffield.
Professor B Williams – University of Nottingham.

THE UNITED STATES

Epidemiological and public health research in the United States during this era is perhaps best viewed in the context of changes that took place during this time in the discipline itself. This was a time when epidemiology in effect came into its own. A community of epidemiologists developed during this time. At least three American epidemiological societies were established – the American Epidemiological Society, the Society for Epidemiological Research and the American College of Epidemiology, in addition to subspecialty epidemiological societies such as the Society for Paediatric Epidemiologic Research. In parallel, there has been an increase in the number of epidemiology journals. Some, such as the American Journal of Epidemiology, which was previously published as the American Journal of Hygiene, predated this period. Others developed *de novo* during this time.

After World War II, major infusions of research funding in the biomedical area became available from the National Institutes of Health (NIH). During this era, major increases in NIH funding for EPHR were also evident. Ultimately, Study Sections were established for reviewing the increasing numbers of proposals submitted for EPHR. In addition, programmes in epidemiology and prevention developed within NIH itself.

An important reflection of the recognition of epidemiology as a discipline is its acceptance as an integral component of both teaching and research in schools of medicine. Many schools now have departments either with epidemiology in their department titles or with other titles such as community or preventive medicine in which epidemiology is a major part of departmental activity. Perhaps even more significant is that within clinical departments, academic staff whose research trajectory is clearly epidemiology are being appointed to tenure tracks and receiving tenure, and these promotions are on the basis of a recognition of EPHR as an important form of biomedical research. Increasing numbers of medical students are now pursuing MD studies, combined either with MPH degrees or with PhD degrees in epidemiology.

Another expression of changes in attitude has been the increasing collaboration of epidemiologists with clinical investigators and basic scientists as seen, for example, in the use of biomarkers in studies of disease aetiology. It is noteworthy that biomarkers are not new to medicine or to epidemiology – for example, phage typing of micro-organisms or serological typing has long been used – but newer advances in molecular biology have expanded the horizons for using newer markers which not only are markers of disease or of exposure but which also can often be localised to specific steps in the pathogenesis of disease and shed light on the mechanisms involved in the development of disease.

A major action in the US was the establishment of the Armed Forces Epidemiology Board in 1941. This was established to investigate "the etiology, epidemiology, prevention and treatment of influenza and other acute epidemic diseases in the Army" and to prepare in peace time for the demands of war. The Board made major contributions to the epidemiology and control of streptococcal disease, the dynamics and prevention of meningococci herd infections and their sequelae, identification of new respiratory viruses and studies leading to vaccine development and their evaluation, such as measles, mumps, Q fever and adenoviruses.

Within the United States federal government, epidemiology has played an increasingly prominent role. For decades after World War II, for example, there was no job classification for epidemiologists and an epidemiologist had to be hired as "statistician." This has clearly changed over time and there are now well recognised classifications for epidemiologists.

There has also been considerable growth of private consulting in epidemiology and in industry-sponsored epidemiology. This includes both the employment of epidemiologists by industry including pharmaceutical manufacturers and the funding by these industries of epidemiological research including randomised trials at academic centres, such as schools of public health and of medicine.

Role of the Epidemiologist

A major difference in opinion has emerged during this time regarding the interface of epidemiology and policy.[1-4] While there is virtually universal agreement that epidemiology has made profound contributions to both public health and clinical policy, there are strong disagreements over the nature of the role of the epidemiologist. Some believe that the role is that of a scientist, pure and simple, without any involvement in policy recommendations and implementations. Others believe, however, that the epidemiologist has an obligation to use his or her findings to participate in the formulation of preventive and other policies, and to help translate EPHR findings into policy.

Methodological Advances

A crucial factor in the explosive growth in epidemiological contributions to public health during this period, in the US as in the UK, has been that of methodological advances. These have been closely coupled with advances in biostatistical methods and with computer advances that have permitted rapid analyses of large amounts of data including the rapid use of statistical models and the use of existing large data sets. The first use of odds ratio was described by Cornfield in 1951.[5] The attributable risk was described by Levin in 1953[6] and the Mantel-Haenszel adjustment was described in 1959.[7] Cornfield published on logistic regression in 1962.[8] New study designs emerged during this period including nested case-control studies and case-cohort studies.

Advances in statistical methodology were, as noted, linked to considerations of design, analysis, and measurement. Good examples of this were considerations of the problems of prospective studies[9] of quantitative methods in the review of epidemiological literature,[10] the analytical methods for case-control studies[11] and the application of these to the evaluation of screening,[12] and elaboration of methods of analysis of survival.[13]

The problems of diagnosis were tackled in a seminal paper by Yerushalmy[14] analysing the variability of interpretation of chest X-ray and the effect of this on diagnosis. He put forward methods of tackling this problem which are still in use. The interpretation of death certificates was comprehensively addressed by Moriyama and his colleagues.[15]

Crucial to many US epidemiological studies over the years has been the careful development of morbidity data based on the Health Interview and Health Examination Surveys which have been undertaken at periodic intervals and have underpinned many of the developments in US health policy, particularly in prevention.[16,17]

EPHR methods have been advanced considerably by the concern for social and cultural factors. Cassel and his group were some of the first leaders in this field in North Carolina,[18] to be followed by Syme and his group in Berkeley, California.[19] The latter profited from the establishment of surveys in a defined county in California, by its then Director of Public Health, Lester Breslow.[20] Francis and Epstein established a defined community study in Tecumseh, Michigan.[21] These defined communities followed the example of Hagerstown, established by Sydenstricker in the 1920s. It is of interest that the direction of investigations in these communities varied. Alameda County studies, for example, have been important in indicating possible, effective preventive strategies, particularly life-style changes. Tecumseh studies concentrated on specific disease entities – for example, cardiovascular disease and infectious disease, particularly acute respiratory and chronic respiratory disease, reflecting the major interests of their staff.

The methods of surveys have been reviewed comprehensively.[22] The first comprehensive discussion of the application and use of genetic data and their utility was published by Neel.[23] Many current studies are based on analysis of serum components collected many years before. The principles of this, and methods of retrieval and storage, were first developed by Paul at Yale, in his studies of polio. A good description is provided by Payne.[24]

Surveillance

The concept of epidemiological surveillance has been greatly advanced during this period. The Centers for Disease Control and Prevention (CDC) have been the main instrument in emphasising the importance of surveillance.[25] Surveillance can be carried out for early disease, for clinically recognizable disease or for risk factors for a disease such as specific exposures. Although surveillance has been shown to be particularly valuable in developing countries, it has clear applications in developed countries as well. One of the major public health triumphs of the twentieth century, the eradication of smallpox,[26–28] was facilitated in part by intensive surveillance and reporting of the disease. This permitted appropriate forces to be marshalled to apply focal immunisation around every local outbreak.

One of the major contributions of epidemiology during this period has been to the study of HIV and AIDS.[29] On 5 June 1981, the Centers for Disease Control and Prevention published five case histories of pneumocystis carinii in young men, all of whom were described as homosexual.[30] Within a year and a half, CDC epidemiologists had developed a working definition of AIDS and identified all of the risk factors. In 1983 CDC issued recommendations for prevention of sexual, drug-related and occupational transmission based on the early EPHR studies and before the cause of AIDS had been identified. Subsequent studies, including the Multi-centred AIDS Cohort Study, have followed populations of men at risk and developed interventions to prevent disease transmission. In addition, the combination of epidemiological data with previous and contemporary work in the basic sciences including molecular biology greatly facilitated the development of new therapeutic interventions for control of the disease.[31–36]

Randomised Trials

This period has been marked by major randomized trials which have made important contributions both to clinical medicine and to public health. Trials in the UK were generally smaller and tighter than in the US where the Public Health Service sponsored larger trials approximating to what might be found in the field. A landmark trial was that of polio vaccine reported in 1955 by Francis.[37] What is now recognized as a classic and pioneering study of screening was the Health Insurance Plan (HIP) controlled trial of breast cancer screening to evaluate mammography and other modalities which was initiated and conducted by Shapiro.[38] The study not only demonstrated the benefits of mammography for women over age 50 years, but the data were also used to analyse racial disparities in deaths from breast cancer.[39] The Lipid Research Clinics Coronary Primary Prevention Trial demonstrated the benefit of reducing cholesterol with cholestyramine in men and has served as a paradigm for prevention trials.[40]

In the treatment area, randomised trials have made major contributions. For example, the trials of different treatments for breast cancer have been noteworthy in determining optimal therapies for women with different stages of breast cancer.[41] The Hypertension Detection and Follow-Up Program elucidated the blood pressure levels at which therapeutic intervention was indicated.[42] During this era, the guidelines established by the Food and Drug Administration were developed, and established the phases of clinical investigation which were needed before a new drug would be approved. In addition, the need for post-marketing surveillance (not a randomised study) were shown to be critical for identifying rare side-effects or those which take a long time to manifest themselves.

Cohort Studies

Cohort studies took several directions during this period. The first type involved the study of cohorts which had had unusual exposures. For example, the Atomic

Bomb Casualty Commission (ABCC), established after World War II and subsequently renamed RERF, conducted studies of the survivors of the Hiroshima and Nagasaki atomic bombings beginning in 1945.[43] These studies provided much needed data regarding radiation epidemiology with a focus on cancers and in particular on leukaemia.[44]

A second type involved the study of populations defined by criteria other than common exposures. An example was Cuyler Hammond's study of cancer among a volunteer population which provided further evidence of the relation of smoking to lung cancer.[45]

A third type established cohorts which were often occupational groups considered likely to participate in long term follow-up. Thus the Physicians' Health Study and the Nurses' Health Study capitalised on groups which were educated and likely to be long-term participants.[46,47] After the initial costs involved in generating the original cohorts, various studies were made possible over subsequent years in a relatively efficient and economical fashion.

One of the most important cohort studies is the Framingham study.[48,49] A variety of hypotheses were tested in a group of 5127 people who were free of CHD at the outset of the study. Many of these hypotheses now seem obvious, mainly as a result of the Framingham study. Issues of weight, smoking, cholesterol and blood pressure were clarified through this cohort study which has been extended to subsequent generations. Perhaps no study has been more rewarding. Much of our fundamental knowledge of the epidemiology of CHD and the potential for its prevention emanated from the Framingham study over a quarter of a century.

Another major cohort study with cross-cultural comparisons was that led by Ancel Keys in which he conducted a multivariate analysis of death and coronary heart disease in seven countries.[50] Among the major findings was the importance of diet and blood pressure and the negligible effect of relative weight or exercise when diet remained a constant.

Case-Control Studies
During the early period discussed previously, the bulk of epidemiological contributions addressed issues of communicable diseases. A major transition occurred during the later period, marked perhaps most prominently by the

Surgeon General's report(s) on smoking beginning in 1964.[51] The question of whether cigarettes were causally related to lung cancer also precipitated a critical examination of the guidelines that could be used for causal inference in non-infectious diseases since the Koch Henle postulates could not be applied.

During this period, it became clear that study designs other than the randomised trial could be applied to the testing of causal inferences regarding an exposure and a disease. Indeed, for ethical and other reasons, randomised trials of putatively toxic agents were not likely to be conducted in human populations. The case-control study attracted increasing prominence as a means for evaluating possible causal relationships, as exemplified by the studies of Wynder and Graham and others on cigarette smoking.[52] Since this design allowed for examining a number of different exposures in relation to a certain disease outcome, the case-control study became a common exploratory type of study and often led to the identification of new relationships. Adenocarcinoma of the vagina and cervix caused by stilboestrol, for example, was identified by Herbst in 1971 through a case-control study and was perhaps the first example of transplacental carcinogenesis.[53]

Other Aetiological Studies
Epidemiology has played a major role in the characterisation of many diseases. Rickettsialpox, for example, was identified by Greenberg in 1947.[54] Among the brilliant achievements of this period was the elucidation of various forms of hepatitis and their epidemiology. Blumberg's work in the discovery of the B-antigen (originally called the Australia antigen) led to his receiving the Nobel Prize.[55,56] The relation of hepatitis B to an increased risk of hepatocellular carcinoma was a major contribution to understanding pathogenesis but also to the potential for preventing this major public health problem.[57]

The relation of slow viruses to chronic diseases was elucidated through a combination of EPHR and laboratory research such as the studies of Kuru by Gajdusek in New Guinea,[58] and subsequent investigations of scrapie and Creutzfeldt-Jakob disease.

An increasing concern with geography as a potential risk factor in disease has benefited from technological progress especially with Global Positioning Systems. Even before these advances, however, geography had proven a valuable factor to consider. For example, the relation of multiple sclerosis to latitude with a north-south gradient was reported by Westlund and Kurland in 1953.[59] Geographical tracing of cases proved to be of great importance in the early days following recognition of AIDS and HIV. The progressive development and geographical spread of the epidemic over time was dramatically shown by spot maps of the United States.

Air Pollution

In 1948 a temperature inversion led to a fog dense with particulates and other contaminants over Donora, Pennsylvania. Of the 14 000 residents, 20 died and 400 required admission to hospital. The investigation that followed has been described as "the first time there was an organised effort to document the health impacts of air pollution in the United States."[60] This episode may well be considered the beginning of air pollution epidemiology in the United States. Studies in this area have attained increasing prominence because of the use of their results by the Environmental Protection Agency and other bodies in setting maximum standards of particulate and other concentrations.

This has led to re-analyses of controversial data such as those of the Harvard Six City Study, to confirm the results used in policy-making.[61]

Occupational Disease

This field was opened up methodologically in the US by Mancuso[62] in studies helped by appropriate analysis of mortality data.[63] The areas of particular note were in the prevalence of respiratory disease in flax workers which used the methods developed in the UK.[64] The other subject of great interest was in the relation of asbestos mining and insulation workers and the development of lung cancer.[65-67] Pleural mesothelioma has been linked to asbestos and not to any other environmental exposure.[68]

An innovative, interesting series of studies on the carpal tunnel syndrome demonstrated the importance of hand-held vibrating tools in the aetiology with high force and repetition increasing the risk 15-fold.[69,70] This has certainly had important implications in the design of work and hand-held tools. Carpal tunnel syndrome is probably quite an important cause of disability.

Epidemiology has been invaluable in many other areas of public health. The Centers for Disease Control and Prevention has listed many of these, including vaccines universally recommended for children, motor vehicle safety, workplace safety, reducing deaths from heart disease and stroke, understanding the hazards of tobacco, enhanced food safety, improved maternal and child health, and control of infectious diseases.

Epidemiology and Health Services Research

Epidemiological methods have found an important place in evaluation, and the use of epidemiology has expanded in health services research and health policy research. Epidemiological approaches have, therefore, been of great interest to those providing insurance coverage for health services and to health maintenance organisations. Epidemiology has been coupled with other disciplines in order to study both effectiveness of care and cost-effectiveness.

A major example of such research was the Rand Health Insurance Experiment in Children published in 1985.[71,72] This large controlled trial investigated the impact of different amounts of co-payment for child health services. Two questions were addressed. The first was whether children use less health care if there is more out-of-pocket cost. This relationship between co-payments and usage was confirmed primarily for surgery and outpatient visits. The second question was whether the health status of children changed with change in the amount of care received. With the outcome measures studied, the authors reported no change. Although the study was subject to methodological criticisms, it was important in demonstrating that the impact of health care on health status could be studied in a rigorous fashion.

The use of EPHR designs and data in health care has a long history in the US, and is often neglected. An early study of quality of care was undertaken by Lembcke shortly after the end of World War II. This was a landmark study, not often quoted by modern authors who have followed on the same lines. Lembcke[73] showed not only variability in the frequency of operations and outcome from a simple operation in different hospitals but, in contrast to many "modern" studies, was based on defined populations rather than only hospital discharges.

The basis of modern evaluation of the quality of health care by considering structure, process and outcome was put forward in a very scholarly fashion by Donabedian.[74,75] An early national study of the outcome of health care resulted[76] from an investigation of a possible association of death following halothane anaesthesia.[77] Breslow[78] and White[79] undertook careful explorations of how epidemiology could contribute to the planning of health services, the former from the standpoint of being responsible for a state population, the latter from a more academic point of view. The contributions of epidemiology and their use were also part of the work of the New York Health Department and its Commissioner, Paul Densen.[80,81]

White was responsible for the organisation of a large international study which examined the use of medical care services of people with similar diagnoses in several countries in the world.[82] It was a carefully executed study which demonstrated that use of hospital facilities is inversely related to the availability and accessibility of ambulatory care. Roemer had previously shown on US admissions that utilisation was associated with availability.[83]

More recently, a group led by Bunker has attempted to analyse the contribution that clinical care now makes to the improvement in health.[84] They claim that now a significant proportion of general health improvement can be attributed to advances in medical care, in contrast to the earlier suggestion of McKeown that most of the changes in health are the result of improvement in nutrition and the environment, including hygiene. Most recently, Anderson and his associates have published a scholarly review of changes in the US health care system which covers some of these issues.[85]

Epidemiology in the Legal and Regulatory Arenas

Epidemiology has assumed a growing importance in other areas as well. Epidemiology plays a major and increasingly critical role in the courts, particularly in toxic tort cases. Many of the rulings involve EPHR evidence and in recent years, rulings by the Supreme Court as in the Daubert case have placed an increasing responsibility upon judges to understand epidemiological and other scientific methods in evaluating whether evidence should be presented to juries. Epidemiologists have therefore taken on new roles in providing education for judges.[86] Beyond the courts, epidemiology is used in risk assessment and environmental regulation.[87] The public health impact of the courts is perhaps most dramatically seen in the landmark lawsuit against the tobacco companies. The public message may perhaps be clearest when translated in monetary damages. Furthermore, in many states, funds obtained through litigation have been invested in EPHR and education.

Disease Control

Having recounted some of the major conceptual and methodological issues tackled during this period, we must also consider the contribution of EPHR to disease control.

Infectious Disease

One of the most feared infections at the beginning of this period was poliomyelitis or infantile paralysis. It is not surprising that a great deal of research was done. Only a few landmark studies have been identified. The importance of different strains of polio virus in different areas was investigated by Paul.[88]

Two groups were involved in the development of a vaccine. Salk was the first to develop an inactivated (killed) vaccine.[89] The evaluation of this has already been mentioned.[37] Inadequate manufacture of a batch of vaccine was associated with an outbreak of paralysis (the Cutter incident). The investigation of this was a classic example of outbreak investigation and of how to handle the situation.[90] The trials of polio vaccine were important in developing methods and many lessons have been learnt.[91,92] The use of killed vaccines was soon superseded by the live vaccine developed by Sabin.[93]

Bacterial infections and their treatment and prevention continued to be important. Streptococcal infection, and subsequent complications, were still rife.[94] Tuberculosis was one of the most important causes of morbidity and led to a series of landmark studies by Comstock and his colleagues.[95] A link to the pre-war period is provided by a study initiated by WH Frost.[96] The importance of bacteria in the development of pyelonephritis, prematurity and their relation to development of chronic disease, including raised blood pressure, was the subject of a series of investigations by Kass in Boston.[97,98]

Acute respiratory infections were the subject of many investigations; most notable were those in defined geographical areas, for example, Tecumseh,[99] or in a defined group of families.[100]

Coronary Heart Disease

As the most important cause of mortality and morbidity, CHD was the subject of an enormous burgeoning of EPHR studies in the post-war period. The studies in Framingham by Dawber and his group[48] and the seven countries study by

Keys[50] have already been mentioned. It is, however, important to consider many other research studies. Of particular note in epidemiology were those by Epstein, one of the first to demonstrate the importance of cultural and ethnic factors influencing the development of disease by comparing populations of Italian background in the US with those of Anglo-Saxon origin, and then developing careful studies of prevalence and incidence in a defined community, Tecumseh.[101]

The need to measure the frequency of cardiovascular findings more accurately led to the development of methods of quantifying reliably ECG findings in the Seven Countries study by Blackburn. These have been beautifully described in a recent book of memoirs.[102]

The investigation of coronary heart disease and associated causes in an occupational group has been the focus of studies by Stamler and his group in Chicago.[103]

The role of exercise and physical fitness in CHD has been extensively studied by Paffenbarger and his group in a series of classical investigations.[104]

The prevention of CHD has already been referred to[40] but an earlier, less successful trial, which was probably one of the first to involve co-operative work in a large number of centres, needs to be remembered.[105] This disease also heralded a series of trials of education in a number of cities – John Farquhar from Stanford was the prime mover of these,[106,107] but other innovative methods were also used in Minnesota.[108]

Blood Pressure
One of the most important risk factors for CHD is raised blood pressure. It is thus not surprising that a series of important, well-conducted studies were done.

The studies by Miall of the distributions of blood pressure in a community in South Wales are discussed earlier in this chapter. Independently and at almost the same time, a similar study was done by Comstock in Georgia.[109] The influence of genetic, cultural and other environmental factors were the subject of several major studies.[110-113]

Data from the Metropolitan Life Insurance Society were used by its chief statistician, Lew, to develop quantitative data on risks.[114] The course and natural history of blood pressure were the subject of both clinical[115] and epidemiological studies.[116–118]

These epidemiological studies led to the first US co-operative study on veterans [119] which provided crucial experience for the much larger trials in general communities described above.[42]

Cancer

As with CHD the number of important studies on the aetiology and prevention of cancer are legion – here we identify only a few of the studies which have had the greatest public impact and illustrate the work of the best investigators.

The National Cancer Institute of the NIH is a very important home to cancer epidemiology in the US. Perhaps of crucial significance in this was the presence of two outstanding researchers from shortly after the end of World War II. Harold Dorn was a statistician who not only worked on methodology but also applied his techniques to a variety of fields, including cancer. He had close personal relations to researchers in the UK – Doll, Bradford Hill and Reid – and shortly after the initiation of the British doctors study he implemented a major long-term study on US veterans which confirmed all of Hill and Doll's findings.[120] In the same Institute, Haenszel began a number of studies on the aetiology of various cancers using data from migrants of different countries and cultures to the USA and comparing cancer incidence between those born in their native country and those born in the United States. His studies, particularly of Japanese, who migrated in two stages, to Hawaii and to the continental United States, were particularly influential in disentangling the role of environment, nutrition, culture and genetics in, for example, gastric cancer.[121] The role of other factors than smoking in cancer of the lung was investigated by Beebe,[122] using the invaluable records of veterans of World War I. The distribution of cancer in the US was monitored continually by the National Cancer Institute and an example was that published by Bailar.[123]

The Department of Epidemiology at Harvard has always had a major interest in cancer epidemiology. Good examples of their work have been the studies of cancer of the breast by MacMahon[124] and of the effects of drugs on the endometrium.[125]

At Johns Hopkins, first Gilliam[126] and later Lilienfeld[127,128] performed several landmark studies.

In New York, Wynder did not limit his investigations to cancer of the lung but used case-control methods on a variety of other cancers to disentangle associations. His studies of cancer of the cervix are a good example.[129] Landrigan was prominent in trying to identify environmental factors – for example, in toxic-waste dumps.[130]

A number of State Health Departments had active EPHR units in the 1960s and early 1970s. One of the most productive of these was in California with Dunn's work on occupational cancers.[131]

Nutrition

We have already mentioned Willett's cohort study of nurses which has been used for the investigation of the association of various dietary components and the occurrence of various conditions, such as colon cancer[47] and breast cancer.[132]

Earlier important studies by Gordon and Scrimshaw were concerned with the importance of diet in relation to illness in early childhood in children in Central America.[133] These investigations have been instrumental in major changes in the policy toward improving child survival in these countries.

Screening

With advances in aetiological knowledge, groups in both the US and UK developed methods of screening for early detection of disease. One of the earliest approaches to considering the methods and theories was a monograph by Thorner and Remein.[134] This has remained a landmark analysis. More recently, other groups have entered the field – for example, McNeil in Boston.[135]

We have already referred to the outstanding trial of breast cancer screening by Shapiro.[38,39] The concept of multi-phasic screening – that is, testing for the presence of several conditions at one visit – was popular at one time, particularly for identifying disease early in pre-paid health plans. Kaiser-Permanente in Oakland, California subjected these to rigorous evaluations.[136,137] In spite of uncertain evidence of benefit, these methods have continued to be used because of popularity with patients.

Psychiatry

Interest and advances in psychiatric epidemiology were at their peak in the early half of this period, aided, perhaps, by the fruition of a number of major population studies which began in the 1940s and earlier.

An early example of how EPHR could be used was the study by Lilienfeld and Pasamanick on events in pregnancy and later development of disease.[138] Shortly thereafter Kramer,[139] a medical statistician, wrote a seminal paper on methods in the field, emphasising the need for non-hospital studies.

The role of social class in mental disease was tackled by Hollingshead and Redlich whose analysis has stood the test of time.[140]

A number of studies in defined communities, such as in New York and its environs, were extremely influential in raising the profile of psychiatric illness.[141-143] The development of psychiatric registers aided the accurate enumeration of the burden of these diseases.[144]

The meaning, measurement and outcome of stress was tackled by Hinkle and Wolff, studies which few now refer to even though they demonstrated current preoccupations.[145]

The misunderstandings (and misconceptions) of the effect of race on psychiatric illness were comprehensively tackled by Pasamanick, almost 40 years ago.[146]

Ageing

With the demographic changes in society it is not surprising that EPHR became involved in a number of studies deliberately focusing on the problems of old age. One of the most interesting hypotheses and analyses was that because of social, environmental and clinical changes, we remain healthy for longer. This was first put forward by Fries[147] in 1980, and has resulted in many studies since that time.[146]

Arthritis

A common condition, arthritis, has been the subject of major studies by two main groups. The approach of Kelsey and her colleagues at Yale and New York and their findings are well summarised in her book.[149] Somewhat earlier, Cobb and his colleagues developed an algorithm for the diagnosis of rheumatoid arthritis [150] whose application was then tested.[151] They also developed other methods and ideas – for example, tackling the problem of transmission.[152]

Congenital Malformations

Of particular note in this field is Ingalls in Philadelphia whose work was crucial, both in quality and in arousing interest in the field.[153] This was followed by an attempt to use vital statistical data to measure incidence.[154] More recently, studies have been published discussing methods of monitoring which are important in the evaluation of changes in medication and treatment during pregnancy.[155]

Dental

This period saw the final analysis of the studies on the benefits of fluoridation established much earlier.[156]

Conclusion

It is important to recognise that this account can only skim the surface of EPHR undertaken in the US in this period. We have limited ourselves to identifying the areas which we believe have resulted in the best work and have been responsible for influencing health policy.

REFERENCES

1 Savitz DA, Poole C, Miller WC. (1999) Reassessing the role of epidemiology in public health. *American Journal of Public Health*, 89: 1158–1161.

2 Jackson LW, Lee NL, Samet JM. (1999) Frequency of policy recommendations in epidemiologic publications. *American Journal of Public Health*, 89: 1206–1211.

3 Krieger N. (1999) Questioning epidemiology: Objectivity, advocacy, and socially responsible science. *American Journal of Public Health*, 89: 1151–1152.

4 Koplan JP, Thacker SB, Lezin NA. (1999) Epidemiology in the 21st century: Calculation, communication and intervention. *American Journal of Public Health*, 89: 1153–1155.

5 Cornfield J. (1951) A method of estimating comparative rates from clinical data. *Journal National Cancer Trust*, 11: 1269–1275.

6 Levin ML. (1953) The occurrence of lung cancer in man. *Acta of the International Union Against Cancer*, 9: 531.

7 Mantel N, Haenszel W. (1959) Statistical aspects of the analysis of data from retrospective studies of disease. *Journal of the National Cancer Trust*, 22: 719–747.

8 Cornfield J. (1962) Joint dependence of risk of coronary heart disease on serum cholesterol and systolic blood pressure: a discriminant function analysis. *Federation Proceedings* 21: 50–61.

9 Dorn H. (1959) Some problems arising in prospective and retrospective studies of aetiology of disease. *New England Journal of Medicine*, 261: 571–579.

10 Greenland S. (1987) Quantitative methods in the review of epidemiologic literature. *Epidemiology Review*, 9: 1–30.

11 Horwitz RI, Feinstein AR. (1978) Alternative analytic methods for case-control studies of estrogens and endometrial cancer. *New England Journal of Medicine*, 299: 1089–1094.

12 Weiss NS. (1994) Application of case-control methods in the evaluation of screening. *Epidemiology Review*, 16: 102–108.

13 Elveback L. (1958) Estimation of survivorship in chronic disease: the "actuarial" method. *Journal of American Statistical Association*, 53: 420–440.

14 Yerushalmy J. (1947) Statistical problems in assessing methods of medical diagnosis; with special reference to x-ray techniques. *Public Health Report*, 62: 1432–1449.

15 Moryiama IM, Baum WS, Haenszel W, Mattison BF. (1958) Inquiry into diagnostic evidence supporting medical certification of death. *American Journal of Public Health*, 48: 1376–1387.

16 US National Health Survey: *Origin and Program of the US National Health Survey*. (1958) Washington, DC: Dept. of Health, Education and Welfare. PHS Publication No. 548–A1.

17 US National Committee on Vital and Health Statistics: *The Analytical Potential of NCHS Data for Health Care Systems* (1973) Washington DC: Health Resources Administration, Dept. of Health, Education and Welfare. Publication No. (HRA) 76–1454.

18 Cassel J, Tyroler HA. (1961) Epidemiological studies of culture change. *Archives of Environmental Health*, 3: 31–39.

19 Berkman LF, Syme SL. (1979) Social Networks, host resistance and mortality: a nine-year follow-up study of Alameda County residents. *American Journal of Epidemiology*, 109: 186.

20 Breslow L. (1965) Alameda and Contra Costa Counties, California. In: *Comparability in International Epidemiology*. Acheson RM (Ed). New York: Milbank Memorial Fund, pp 317–325.

21 Francis T, Epstein FH. (1965) Tecumseh, Michigan. Ibid., pp 333–344.

22 Kelsey JL, Thompson WD, Evans AS. (1986) *Methods in Observational Epidemiology*. Oxford: Oxford University Press.

23 Neel JV, Shaw MW, Schull WJ (Eds). (1965) *Genetics and the epidemiology of chronic disease*. Washington, DC: Dept. of Health, Education and Welfare. PHS Publication No. 1163.

24 Payne AM-M. (1965) Serum surveys. In: *Comparability in International Epidemiology*. Acheson RM (Ed). New York: Milbank Memorial Fund, pp 345–350.

25 Langmuir AD. (1963) The surveillance of communicable diseases of national importance. *New England Journal of Medicine*, 268: 182–192.

26 Henderson DA. (1976) Surveillance smallpox. *International Journal of Epidemiology*, 5: 19–28.

27 Foege WH, Millar JD, Henderson DA. (1975) Smallpox eradication in West and Central Africa. *Bulletin of the World Health Organisation*, 52: 209–222.

28 Fenner F, Henderson DA, Arita I, et al. (1988) *Smallpox and its Eradication*. Geneva: World Health Organisation.

29 Communicable Disease Center. HIV and AIDS – United States 1981–2001. (2001) *Morbidity and Mortality Weekly Report*, 50: 430–439.

30 Gottlieb MS, Schroff R, Schanker HM, et al. (1981) Pneumocystis carinii pneumonia and mucosal candidiasis in previously healthy homosexual men, evidence of a new aquired immunodeficiency. *New England Journal Medicine*, 305: 1425–1431.

31 Essex ME. (1997) Origin of acquired immunodeficiency syndrome. In: *AIDS: Biology, Diagnosis, Treatment and Prevention*. De Vita VT Jr, Hellman S, Rosenberg SA, Curran J, et al (Eds). 4th edition. New York: Lippincott Raven.

32 Detels R, Vissher BR, Faley JL. (1987) Predictors of AIDS in young homosexual men in a high risk area. *International Journal of Epidemiology*, 16: 271–276.

33   Dean M, Carrington M, Winkler C, et al. (1996) Genetic restriction of HIV-1 infection and progression to Aids by a deletion allele of the CKR5 structural gene. Haemophilia growth and development study. Multicenter AIDS cohort study. San Francisco City Cohort. ALIVE Study. *Science*, 273: 1856–1862.

34   Kaslow R, Ostrow D, Detels R, et al. (1987) The Multicentre Aids cohort study: national, organisation and selected characteristics of the participants. *American Journal of Epidemiology*, 126: 310–318.

35   Jacobsen L, Yamashita T, Detels R, et al. (1999) Impact of potent antiretroviral therapy on the incidence of Kaposi's sarcoma and non-Hodgkins lymphomas among HIV-I infected individuals. Multicenter Aids Cohort Study. *Journal Aids* Suppl 1: 534–541.

36   Quinn TC, Fauci AS. (1998) The Aids epidemic: Demographic aspects, population biology, and virus evolution. In: *Emerging Infections*. Krause RM (Ed). San Diego, London: Academic Press, pp 327–363.

37   Francis T, Napier RB, Voight FM. (1955) Evaluation of 1954 field trials of poliomyelitis vaccine. *American Journal of Public Health*, 45: 5.

38   Shapiro S, Venet W, Strax P, et al. (1971) Ten to fourteen year effect of screening on breast cancer mortality. *Journal of the National Cancer Institute*, 69: 349–355.

39   Shapiro S, Venet W, Strax P, et al. (1982) Prospects for eliminating racial differences in breast cancer survival rates. *American Journal of Public Health*, 72: 1142–1145.

40   Lipid Research Clinics Program. The Lipid Research Clinics Coronary Primary Prevention Trial. Results: I. Reduction in incidence of coronary heart disease. *JAMA*, 251: 351–364.

41   Fisher B, Redmond C, Fisher ER, et al. (1985) Ten-year results of a randomized clinical trial comparing radical mastectomy and total mastectomy with or without radiation. *New England Journal of Medicine*, 312: 674–681.

42 Hypertension Detection and Follow-up Program Co-operative Group. (1979) Five Year Findings of the Hypertension Detection and Follow-up Program. I. Reduction of Mortality in persons with high blood pressure, including mild hypertension. *JAMA*, 242: 2562–2571.

43 ABCC-RERF study of Hiroshima and Nagasaki. (1985) *National Cancer Institute Monograph*, 67: 53–58.

44 Bizzozero OJ, Johnson KG, Ciocco A, et al. (1966) Radiation-related leukemia in Hiroshima and Nagasaki, 1946–1964. I. Distribution, incidence and appearance time. *New England Journal of Medicine*, 274: 1095–1101.

45 Hammond EC, Horn D. (1958) Smoking and death rates – Report on 44 months of follow-up of 187,783 men. Part I Total mortality. Part II Death rates by cause. *JAMA*, 166: 1159–1172; 1294–1308.

46 The Steering Committee of the Physicians' Health Study Research Group. Final report on the aspirin component of the ongoing Physicians' Health Study. (1989)*New England Journal of Medicine*, 321: 129–135.

47 Willett WC, Stampfer MJ, Colditz GA, et al. (1990) Relation of meat, fat and fibre intake to the risk of colon cancer in a prospective study among women. *New England Journal of Medicine*, 323: 1664–1672.

48 Dawber TR, Kannel WB, Lyell LP. (1963) An approach to longitudinal studies in a community: The Framingham Study. *Annals of the New York Academy of Sciences*, 107: 539–556.

49 Kannel WB. (1983) *Prevention of Coronary Heart Disease: Practical Management of the risk factors*. Kaplan NM, Stamler J (Eds). Philadelphia, PA: WB Saunders Co.

50 Keys A. (1980) *Seven Countries: A Multivariate Analysis of Death and Coronary Heart Disease*. Cambridge, MA: Harvard University Press.

51 Report of the Advisory Committee to the Surgeon General of the Public Health Services. (1964) *Smoking and Health*. Washington, DC: Public Health Service. Publication No. 1103.

52 Wynder EL, Graham EA. (1950) Tobacco smoking as a possible etiologic factor in bronchogenic carcinoma: A study of six hundred and eighty four proven cases. *JAMA*, 143: 329–336.

53 Herbst AL, Ulfeder H, Poskanzer DC. (1971) Adenocarcinoma of the vagina: Association of maternal stillbestrol therapy with tumor appearance in young women. *New England Journal of Medicine*, 284: 878–881.

54 Greenberg M, Pellitteri OJ, Jellison WL. (1947) Rickettsialpox. A newly recognised Rickettsial Disease. *American Journal of Public Health*, 37: 860–868.

55 Blumberg BS, Alter HJ, Visnisch S. (1965) A "new" antigen in leukemia sera. *JAMA*, 191: 541–546.

56 Prince AM. (1968) An antigen detected in the blood during the incubation period of infectious hepatitis. *Procedings of the National Academy of Sciences of the USA*, 60: 814–821.

57 Beasley RP, Hwong LY, Lin CC, Chicu CS. (1981) Hepatocellular carcinoma and hepatitis B virus. A prospective study of 22,207 men in Taiwan. *Lancet*, 2: 1129–1133.

58 Gajdusek DC, Zigas V. (1959). Kuru. Clinical, pathological and epidemiological study of an acute progressive degenerative disease of the central nervous system among natives of the Eastern Highlands of New Guinea. *American Journal of Medicine*, 26: 442–469.

59 Westlund K, Kurland LT. (1953) Studies on Multiple Sclerosis in Winnipeg, Manitoba and New Orleans, Louisiana. *American Journal of Hygiene*, 57: 380–407.

60 Schrenk HH, Heimann H, Clayton GD, Gafafer WM. (1949) Air Pollution in Donora, PA. *US Public Health Bulletin 306*.

61 Dockery DW, Pope CA. (1994) Acute respiratory effects of particulate air pollution. *Annual Review of Public Health*, 15: 107–132.

62 Mancuso TF, Coulter EJ. (1959) Methods of studying the relation of employment and long term illness – cohort analysis. *American Journal of Public Health*, 49: 1525–1536.

63 Guralnick L. (1963) Mortality by occupation level and cause of death among men aged 20–64 years of age. United States, 1950. *Vital Statistics Special Reports*, 53: 439–612.

64 Ferris BG, Anderson DO, Burgess WA. (1962) Prevalence of respiratory disease in a flax mill in the United States. *British Journal of Industrial Medicine*, 19: 180–185.

65 Enterline PE. (1965) Mortality among asbestos products workers in the United States. *Annals of the New York Academy of Sciences*, 132: 156–165.

66 Selikoff IJ, Churg J, Hammond EC. (1964) Asbestos exposure and neoplasia. *JAMA*, 188: 22.

67 Selikoff IJ, Hammond EC, Churg J. (1968) Asbestos exposure, smoking and neoplasia. *JAMA*, 204: 106–112.

68 Craighead JE, Mossman BT. (1982) The pathogenesis of asbestos-related diseases. *New England Journal of Medicine*, 306: 1446–1455.

69 Cummings K, Maizlish N, Rudolph L, Durvin K, et al. (1989) Occupational disease surveillance: carpal tunnel syndrome. *Mortality and Morbidity Weekly Reports*, 38: 485–489.

70 Franklin GM. (1994) Peripheral Neuropathy. In: *Handbook of Neuroepidemiology*. Gorelick PB, Maalter A (Eds). New York: Marcel Dekker, pp 381–405.

71 Leibowitz A, Manning WG, Keeleer EB, et al .(1985) Effect of cost sharing on the use of medical services by children: Interim results from a randomised controlled trial. *Pediatrics*, 75: 942–951.

72 Valdez RB, Brook RH, Rogers WH, et al. (1985) Consequences of cost sharing for children's health. *Pediatrics*, 75: 952–961.

73   Lembkce P. (1952) Increasing the quality of medical care through vital statistics based on hospital service areas: I. Comparative study of append-ectomy rates. *American Journal of Public Health*, 42: 276–286.

74   Donabedian A. (1973) *Aspects of medical care administration specifying requirements for health care*. Cambridge, MA: Harvard University Press.

75   Donabedian A. (1966) Evaluating the quality of medical care. *Milbank Memorial Fund Quart*erly, 44: 166–206.

76   National Research Council. (1969) *The National Halothane Study: a study of the possible association between halothane anaesthesia and post operative hepatic necrosis*. Bunker JP, Forest WH, Mosteller F, Vandam LD (Eds). Washington, DC: National Institute of Health, National Institute of General Medical Sciences, US General Post Office.

77   Stanford Center for Health Care Research. (1976) *Study of Institutional Differences in Post-Operative Mortality*. National Research Council Publication 250940. Assembly of Life Sciences, Nat. Institute of General Medical Sciences Bureau of Health Services Research, Dept. of Health, Education and Welfare, 1–266 and 1–496.

78   Breslow L. (1958) The evaluation of health needs and services in California by the epidemiological method. In: *Recent Studies in Epidemiology*. Pemberton J, Willard H (Eds). Oxford: Blackwell.

79   White KL, Henderson MM. (1976) *Epidemiology as a Fundamental Science. Its uses in Health Service Planning, Administration and Evaluation*. Oxford: Oxford University Press.

80   Jones EW, Densen PM, Altman I, et al. (1974) HIP incentive reimbursement experiment: utilization and costs of medical care, 1969 and 1970. *Social Security Bulletin*, 39: No. 12.

81   Densen PM. (1976) Epidemiologic contributions to health services research. *American Journal of Epidemiology*, 104: 478–488.

82 Kohn R, White KL. (1976) *Health Care: An international study*. Oxford: Oxford University Press.

83 Roemer ML. (1961) Bed supply and hospital utilisation: a national experiment. *Hospitals*, 1: 36–42.

84 Bunker JP, Frazier HS, Mosteller F. (1994) Improving health: measuring effects of medical care. *Milbank Quarterly*, 72: 225–258.

85 Anderson JM, Rice TH, Kominski GF. (2000) *Changing the US Health Care System. Key issues in Health Services, Policy and Management*. 2nd edition. San Francisco, CA: Josey-Bass.

86 Green M, Freedman M, Gordis L. (2000) *Reference Guide on Epidemiology, Reference Manual on Scientific Evidence*. 2nd edition. Washington, DC: Federal Judicial Center.

87 Samet JM, Schnatter R, Gibb H. (1998) Invited Commentary: Epidemi-ology and risk assessment. *American Journal of Epidemiology*, 148: 929–936.

88 Paul JR, Melnick JL, Riordan JT. (1952) Comparative neutralising antibody patterns to lansing (type 2) poliomyelitis virus in different populations. *American Journal of Hygiene*, 56: 232–251.

89 Salk JE. (1955) Considerations in the preparation and use of poliomyelitis virus vaccine. *JAMA*, 158: 1239–1248.

90 Nathanson N, Langmuir AD. (1963) The Cutter incident. Poliomyelitis following fomaldehyde inactivated polio virus vaccine in the United States in the spring of 1955. *American Journal of Hygiene*, 78: 16–28.

91 Monto AS. (1999) Francis Field Trial of inactivated Polio Vaccine. Background and lessons for today. *Epidemiology Review*, 21: 7–23.

92 Francis T Jr., Napier JA, Voight RB, et al. (1957) Evaluation of the 1954 field trial of poliomyelitis vaccine: final report. Ann Arbor, MI: Edward Brothers.

93 Sabin AB. (1949) *Epidemiologic patterns of poliomyelitis in different parts of the world*. Conference paper at International Polio Conference. Philadelphia, PA. pp 3–33.

94 Feinstein AR, et al. (1959) A controlled study of three methods of prophylaxis against streptococcal infection in a population of rheumatic children. *New England Journal of Medicine*, 260: 697–702.

95 Comstock GW. (1949) Tuberculosis studies in Muscogee County, Georgia. I Community wide tuberculosis research. *Public Health Report*, 64: 259–263.

96 Zeidberg LD, Gass RS, Dillon A, Hutsheson RH. (1963) The Williamson County Tuberculosis study. A 24-year epidemiologic study. *American Review of Respiratory Disease*, 87: No. 3 part 2.

97 Kass EH. (1957) Bacteriuria and the diagnosis of infections of the urinary tract. *Archives of Internal Medicine*, 100: 709–714.

98 Kass EH, Savage W, Santamarina BAG. (1965) The significance of bacteriuria in preventive medicine, In: *Progress in Pyelonephritis*. Kass EH (Ed). Philadelphia, PA. Davis FA & Co, 3–10.

99 Monto AS, Lim SK. (1974) The Tecumseh study of respiratory illness. VI Frequency and relationship between outbreaks of coronavirus infection. *Journal of Infectious Disease*, 129: 271–276.

100 Dingle JH, Badger GF, Jordan WS. (1964) *Illness in the Home. A Study of 25,000 Illnesses in a Group of Cleveland Families*. Cleveland, OH: The Press of Western Reserve University.

101 Epstein FH. (1965) The epidemiology of coronary heart disease – a review. *Journal of Chronic Disease*, 18: 735–774.

102 Blackburn H. (1995) On the trail of heart attacks in seven countries. Private publication.

103 Shekelle RB, Shryock AM, Paul O, et al. (1981) Diet, serum cholesterol and death from coronary heart disease: The Western Electric study. *New England Journal of Medicine*, 304: 65–70.

104 Kohl HW, Powell KE, Gordon NF, et al. (1992) Physical activity, physical fitness and sudden cardiac death. *Epidemiology Review*, 14: 37–58.

105 Multiple risk factor intervention trial group. (1977) Statistical design consideration in the NHLI multiple risk factors intervention trial. (MRFIT) *Journal of Chronic Disease*, 20: 261–275.

106 Farquhar J, Maccoby N, Wood PD, Alexander JK, et al. (1977) Community education for cardiovascular health. *Lancet*, 1 : 1192–1195

107 Farquhar J, Fortmann SP, et al. (1990) Effects of community wide education on cardiovascular disease risk factors. The Stanford Five-City project. *JAMA*, 264: 359–365.

108 Luepker RV, Murray DM, Jacobs R, Mittelmark MB, et al. (1994) Community education for cardiovascular disease prevention: risk factor changes in the Minnesota Heart Health Program. *American Journal of Public Health*, 84: 1383–1393.

109 Comstock GW. (1957) An epidemiologic study of blood pressure levels in a biracial community in the southern United States. *American Journal of Hygiene*, 65: 271–315.

110 Feinleib M, Garrison MS, Borhani N, Rosenman R, et al. (1975) Studies of hypertension in twins. In: *Epidemiology and Control of Hypertension*. Paul O (Ed). New York: Stratton International, pp 3–20.

111 Cassel J. (1975) Studies of hypertension in migrants. Ibid., pp 41–62.

112 Tyroler HA, Heyden S, Hames CG. (1975) Weight and hypertension: Evans County Study of Blacks and Whites. Ibid., pp 177–206.

113   Stamler J, Berkson DM, Dyer A, Lepper MH, et al. (1975) Relationship of multiple variables to blood pressure. Four Chicago epidemiologic studies. Ibid., pp 307–358.

114   Lew EA. (1967) Blood pressure and mortality – life insurance experience. In: *The Epidemiology of Hypertension*. Stamler J, Stamler R, Pullman TN (Eds). New York: Grune and Stratton, pp 392–397.

115   Paul O. (1967) The Natural History of Hypertension. Ibid., pp 365–374.

116   Winkelstein W, Kantor S. (1967) Some observations on the relationship between age, sex and blood pressure. Ibid., pp 70–81.

117   Chapman JM, Borun ER, Massey FJ, et al. (1967) Blood pressure distributions in the Los Angeles Heart Study 1950–1963. Ibid., pp 98–100.

118   Epstein FH, Eckoff RD. (1967) The Epidemiology of High Blood Pressure – geographic distributions and aetiological factors. Ibid., pp 155–166.

119   Freis ED. (1975) The Veterans Administration Co-operative study. In: *Epidemiology and Control of Hypertension*. Paul O (Ed). New York: Stratton Intercontinental, pp 449–460.

120   Kahn HA. (1966) The Dorn study of smoking and mortality among US veterans. Report on eight and a half years of observations. In: *Epidemiological Approaches to the Study of Cancer and Other Chronic Diseases*. Haenszel W (Ed). National Cancer Institute, Monograph 19. Washington, DC: US Government Printing Office, pp 1–125.

121   Haenszel W, Kurihara M. (1968) Studies of Japanese migrants. I. Mortality from cancer and other diseases among Japanese in the United States. *Journal of the National Cancer Institute*, 40: 43–68.

122   Beebe GW. (1960) Lung cancer in World War I veterans: possible relation to mustard-gas injury and 1918 influenza pandemic. *Journal of the National Cancer Institute*, 25: 1231–1252.

123 Bailar JC III. (1969) The Third National Cancer Survey. *Cancer*, 19: 228–231.

124 MacMahon B. (1958) Cohort fertility and increasing breast cancer incidence. *Cancer*, 11: 250–254.

125 Ziehl HK, Finkle WD. (1975) Increased risk of endometrial carcinoma among users of conjugated oestrogens. *New England Journal of Medicine*, 293: 1167–1170.

126 Gilliam AG. (1954) A note on evidence relating to the incidence of primary liver cancer among the Bantu. *Cancer Institute*, 15: 195–199.

127 Lilienfeld AM. (1964) The relationship of bladder cancer to smoking. *American Journal of Public Health*, 54: 1864–1875.

128 Lilienfeld AM, Gifford A. (Eds). (1966) *Chronic Diseases and Public Health*. Baltimore, MD: Johns Hopkins Press.

129 Wynder EL, Cornfield J, Schroff PD, Doraiswami KR, et al. (1954) A study of environmental factors in carcinoma of the cervix. *American Journal of Obstetrics and Gynaecology*, 68: 1016–1052.

130 Landrigan PJ. (1983) Epidemiologic approaches to persons with exposures to waste chemicals. *Environmental Health Perspectives*, 48: 93–97.

131 Dunn JE, Weir JM. (1965) Cancer experience of several occupational groups followed prospectively. *American Journal of Public Health*, 55: 1367–1375.

132 Willett WC, Hunter DJ, Stampfer NJ, Colditz G, et al. (1992) Dietary fat and fibre in relation to breast cancer. *JAMA*, 268: 2037–2044.

133 Gordon JE, Scrimshaw NS. (1965) Nutrition and the diarrhoeas of early childhood in the tropics. In: *Comparability in International Epidemiology*. Acheson RM (Ed). New York: Milbank Memorial Fund, pp 233–239.

134   Thorner RM, Remein QR. (1961) Principles and procedures in the evaluation of screening for disease. *Public Health Monograph*, No.67 (Public Health Service Publication No. 846).

135   McNeil BJ, Adelstein SJ. (1976) Determining the value of diagnostic and screening tests. *Journal of Nuclear Medicine*, 17: 439–448.

136   Collen MF. (1973) Multi-phasic check-up evaluation study 4. Preliminary cost-benefit analysis for middle-aged men. *Preventive Medicine*, 2: 236–246.

137   Friedman GD. (1978) Effects of MHTS on patients. pp 531–549. In: *Multi-phasic Health Testing Services*. Collen MF (Ed). New York: Wiley.

138   Lilienfeld AM, Pasamanick B, Rogers M. (1955) Relationship between pregnancy experience and the development of certain neuropsychiatric disorders in childhood. *American Journal of Public Health*, 45: 637–643.

139   Kramer M. (1957) A discussion of the concepts of incidence and prevalence as related to epidemiologic studies of mental disorders. *American Journal of Public Health*, 47: 826–840.

140   Hollingshead AB, Redlich FC. (1958) *Social Class and Mental Illness*. New York: Wiley.

141   Srole L, Langner TS, Michael ST, Opler MK, et al. (1962) *Mental Health in the Metropolis: the Mid-town Manhattan Study*. Vols I and II. New York: McGraw Hill.

142   Gruenberg EM. (1965) A review of mental health in the metropolis: the mid-town Manhattan study. *International Journal of Psychiatry*, 1: 77–86.

143   Leighton DC, Harding JS, Macklin DB, et al. (1963) Psychiatric findings of the Stirling County Study. *American Journal of Psychiatry*, 119: 1021–1026.

144   Bahn AK, Gardner EA, Alltop L, Knatterud GL, et al. (1966) Admission and prevalence rates for psychiatric facilities in four register areas. *American Journal of Public Health*, 56: 2033–2051.

145 Hinkle LE, Wolff HG. (1957) The nature of man's adaptation to his total environment and the relation of this to illness. *Archive of International Medicine*, 99: 442–460.

146 Pasamanick B (Ed). (1963) Some misconceptions concerning differences in the racial prevalence of mental disease. *American Journal of Orthopsychiatry*, 33: 72–86.

147 Fries JF. (1980) Ageing, natural death and the compression of morbidity. *New England Journal of Medicine*, 303: 130–155.

148 Brody JA, Schneider EC. (1986) Diseases and disorders of ageing: an hypothesis. *Journal of Chronic Disease*, 39: 871–876.

149 Kelsey JL, Pastides H, Bisbee G. (1978) *Musculo-Skeletal Disorders. Their Frequency of Occurrence and Their Impact on the Population of the United States.* New York: Prodist.

150 Cobb S, Merchant WR, Warren JR. (1955) An epidemiologic look at the problem of classification in the field of arthritis. *Journal of Chronic Disorders*, 2: 50–54.

151 Ropes MW, Bennett GA, Cobb S et al. (1957) Proposed diagnostic criteria for rheumatoid arthritis. Report of a study conducted by a committee of the American Rheumatism Association. *Journal of Chronic Disease*, 5: 630–635.

152 Cobb S, Harburg E, Tabor J, Hunt P, et al. (1967) The intrafamilial transmission of rheumatoid arthritis. I Design II An interview measure. *Journal of Chronic Disease*, 22: 195–215.

153 Ingalls TH. (1960) Prenatal human ecology. *American Journal of Public Health*, 50: 50–54.

154 Gittelsohn AM, Milham S. (1965) Vital record incidence of congenital malformations in New York State. In: *Genetics and the Epidemiology of Chronic Disease.* Neel JV, et al. (Eds). PHS Publication No. 1163. Washington, DC: Public Health Service.

155   Holtzman NE, Khoury MJ. (1986) Monitoring for congenital malformations. *Annual Review of Public Health*, 7: 237–266.

156   Ast DB, Schlesinger E. (1956) The conclusion of a ten year study of water fluoridation. *American Journal of Public Health*, 46: 265–271.

4. Where is Epidemiological Public Health Research Done and Who Pays?

THE UNITED KINGDOM

To attempt to understand research in EPHR, it is important to have some knowledge of the places where it is carried out. Almost all such research is undertaken in universities or research establishments. In the United Kingdom there are no significant private or commercial enterprises which undertake EPHR. Some research is done by service organisations such as local or central health departments. Funding for research is from either governmental, local or central sources, or from private foundations. Unfortunately, it has not been possible to obtain meaningful figures for research expenditures on EPHR. The categories listed are often so confused or overlapping that it is impossible to separate various roles and contributions. Funding agencies do not keep records in a way that enables analysis to be carried out.

Universities

1919–1939

In this time period there were 16 universities in the United Kingdom which had medical schools or medical faculties. Of the 15 outside London, all but Dundee (St Andrews), Oxford, Manchester and Birmingham had academic departments concerned with public health/epidemiology. In England, five universities with an academic department – Newcastle, Liverpool, Leeds, Sheffield and Bristol – had joint appointments with the local city health department – usually the professor was also the Medical Officer of Health. Presumably some of the teaching and research was done by his health department staff but we could only find one named individual in each university. Cambridge, by contrast, in this period had one named, full-time academic in the field – the exact title of the post varied but ended with "human ecology".

In contrast, Wales had a professor and up to four named academic full-time appointments during this period. Three of the four Scottish universities – Aberdeen, Glasgow and Edinburgh – had a full-time professor almost continuously. Aberdeen also had a full-time senior lecturer, while Glasgow and Edinburgh usually also had two senior lecturers.

Queen's University, Belfast had a full-time professor and a senior lecturer throughout this period.

In London the situation was quite different. Of the 12 medical schools only one had a part-time appointment (University College). The London School of Tropical Medicine changed its title and role to London School of Hygiene and Tropical Medicine and began the teaching of post-graduate public health and epidemiology as well as research in these subjects in 1928.

When the joint School started in 1928, its Department of Epidemiology and Vital Statistics had one professor (Major Greenwood) and three others who were either joint appointments with Bacteriology and Immunology or attached workers from the Medical Research Council (for example, Austin Bradford Hill). The Department of Bacteriology and Immunology was headed by a professor (WWC Topley) and had two other full-time academics (including GS Wilson). Much of the published research was done jointly by these two departments. The Department of Public Health was headed by Professor WW Jameson. By 1929 this department had, in addition, an Assistant Director (Parkinson) and five lecturers. The Department of Bacteriology had expanded to a professor, two lecturers, a demonstrator, and Dr GS Wilson was promoted to reader. Epidemiology had two university lecturers (full-time) and four attached Medical Research Council workers. Subsequently, the Public Health Department added up to 22 special lecturers, whose primary employment was as Medical Officers of Health, His Majesty's Inspectors of Factories, or Medical Officers in the Ministry of Health.

These complements of one professor with three to five full-time academics in each of these departments continued until 1948. Obviously, there were changes – Bradford Hill, for example, became a university reader in 1934. There was one interesting appointment in 1932 to the Department of Epidemiology, Dr LWG Malcolm as lecturer in Racial Hygiene. He left in 1934.

The situation of public health in universities needs to be put in context. In general, there were relatively few full-time academic appointments in medicine or other clinical disciplines. Professors were appointed in "theoretical" subjects such as anatomy, physiology, and pathology. Only a very few universities had a full-time Professor of Medicine before 1919 in England, although the Scottish universities had such posts. Academic appointments in clinical subjects began to be made only after the war, in 1919, and even by 1960 not all medical schools in London had a Professor of Medicine. It was the Medical Research Council which stimulated the appointment of full-time clinical academics. The "provincial" universities in England were ahead of the University of London and its medical schools. Only in Scotland and Northern Ireland was medicine recognised as a subject for academic enquiry. In London, in particular, clinical medicine was taught largely by clinicians in the voluntary (teaching) hospitals and full-time academic appointments were rare.

1946–1969

After World War II the academic establishment expanded. Not unexpectedly, however, the universities (Schools) with a "history" of public health expanded more rapidly than the others.

Belfast had a professor and six lecturer/senior lecturer posts, and the four Scottish universities now all had full-time professors with two and up to six supporting lecturer posts. Cardiff had a professor, three senior lecturers and three lecturers. Oxford now had a professor (or reader) and one other, Cambridge three others. Sheffield, Birmingham and Bristol had full-time professors, each with one supporting lecturer. Newcastle, Manchester, Liverpool and Leeds continued with part-time professors. The subject was called Social Medicine from 1942 in Oxford (Ryle), Birmingham (McKeown), Trinity College, Dublin (Jessop), Social and Industrial Medicine in Sheffield, and Social and Preventive Medicine in Belfast.[1] The nomenclature of the subject has changed many times over the past 100 years, even if the content remains the same.[2]

In London, the Medical Schools continued to lag behind in academic appointments in epidemiology and public health. Several – the Royal Free Hospital, the London Hospital and University College Hospital – had part-time appointments jointly with the London School of Hygiene and Tropical Medicine or the Medical Research Council. Only St Thomas's created a full-time senior lecturer post in 1961/2 with two supporting lecturers in 1963/4. Guy's also created a full-time post of senior lecturer in 1969, having had, for a short period (1961–2), a reader (RM Acheson). Some Schools, such as those at King's College Hospital, Westminster Hospital, and Charing Cross Hospital, had no specific posts while others rapidly followed the lead of St. Thomas's.

St Mary's appointed a senior lecturer (Dr GA Rose) jointly with the Department of Epidemiology at the London School of Hygiene in the mid 1960s. The Middlesex began moves to create a Department in the late 1960s, and appointed a senior lecturer (Dr G Kazantzis). It was the first to establish a Chair in 1971 (Prof D Miller) rather than conferring a personal title of Professor.

The attitude of London medical schools to academic appointments was not limited to epidemiology and public health. Some Schools only appointed their first Professor of Medicine or Surgery in the mid to late 1950s and some had no such appointment until the end of this time period. Similarly in Child Health there was only one professor (Moncrieff) at Great Ormond Street and one in psychiatry (Aubrey Lewis) at the Maudsley Hospital.

The University of London excused lack of expenditure on academic epidemiology and public health by emphasising that it funded academic appointments at the London School of Hygiene – there were two full-time professors (Bradford Hill and Mackintosh, and later Walton) as well as a full-time reader or senior lecturer and several part-time appointments. The school also housed a number of individual Medical Research Council workers as well as the Medical Research Council Statistical Epidemiological Research Unit.

It is not the purpose of this book to describe the evolution of academic epidemiology and public health in London or elsewhere in detail; it is, however, important to appreciate what limited manpower resources were available.

1970–Present Day
The staffing of public health university departments has expanded greatly since 1970. In 1992 Clarke and Kurinzcuk,[3] on behalf of all academic departments, reviewed the current staffing and found that there were now 121 medically qualified academics, 36 statisticians, 23 social scientists and 36 other staff employed. Thirty of these were professors, 99 readers or senior lecturers and 87 lecturers. By 1992 every medical school in the UK had at least one academic member of staff and most had more than this bare minimum. Between 1968 and 1970 three new medical schools were started: Southampton, Leicester and Nottingham. Each of these schools had a Foundation Professor of Public Health (or equivalent) and all had adequate supporting staff.

Medical Research Council

There are two major accounts of the Medical Research Council since its foundation as the Medical Research Committee in 1913.[4,5]

Since its inception, the Medical Research Council has played an important role in the funding and promotion of EPHR. It is not appropriate to describe the history of the MRC in this book but we will discuss and describe its role in sustaining EPHR.

The MRC supports research through a system of project and programme grants and support of central research facilities The latter include the National Institute of Medical Research and later the Medical Research Council Clinical Research Centre at Northwick Park Hospital (now defunct). It also supports individual research units, individual researchers, including senior career awards and training fellowships. The balance and location of these has changed over time. Although the MRC's self-professed aim from the 1920s was primarily to promote basic biomedical research, it has always also played a very important role in the more applied public health field.

From the start the MRC supported a statistical department. They saw its function as being "(a) to undertake statistical research into problems of epidemiology and the like, and (b) to advise and assist other research workers in applying statistical treatment to a wide variety of data".[4] Dr John Brownlee was first appointed to this department and was joined by Dr Major Greenwood who moved from the Lister Institute and Ministry of Health in 1920. After Brownlee's death in 1927 the department was moved, under Greenwood, to the London School of Hygiene, where it was the core of the nascent Department of Epidemiology.

The MRC continued to support the work at the London School of Hygiene through combined staff appointments. When Dr (later Sir) Austin Bradford Hill succeeded Greenwood as Professor it became a separately identified Statistical Research Unit, with Bradford Hill as honorary director. On his retirement in 1965 he was succeeded by Dr (later Sir) Richard Doll and the unit became an entirely separate entity with other accommodation found by the Council. In 1970 most of the staff were transferred to the new Clinical Research Centre for its Division of Epidemiology and Medical Care Unit at Northwick Park

Hospital under the direction of Dr TW Meade. The statistical (and computing) unit developed a separate existence at the Clinical Research Centre, and later in Cambridge.

The unit concept took off after 1945. The major units specifically related to EPHR were the Pneumoconiosis Research Unit established in 1945,[6] Social Medicine (first at the Central Middlesex Hospital and then at the London Hospital), Epidemiology (South Wales) and Psychiatry (Edinburgh). In addition the Medical Research Council was extremely interested in nutrition and has funded the Dunn Laboratory in Cambridge since 1926.

Landsborough Thompson [4] gives a factual account of the areas of research in which the MRC was particularly active. The foundation of the MRC was, at first, linked to the National Insurance system and tuberculosis. As a result in 1914, 46% of its expenditure of £19 350 was on tuberculosis, 18% on rickets, and 11% on the health aspects of milk. The MRC played an important role in supporting the war effort during World War I, for example, by the investigation of methods of prevention of "trench foot" and the treatment of the effects of gas warfare. The organisation was thus in a "politically" advantageous position to influence medical research policy after the war.

Although the MRC continued to support research on the major health problems of the day, and made important contributions to their solution, the balance shifted somewhat from practical to theoretical or experimental work.

One of the main areas of interest in the early years was in nutrition. The MRC "moved rapidly to the forefront in nutritional research at an international level but scientific data were used to reinforce current prejudices regarding working class ignorance and inefficiency and explains that where steps were taken to apply the newer knowledge of nutrition, the results were either irrelevant or counter-productive."[5] This contrasted with the work of Boyd Orr[7] from the Rowett Research Institute and with that of a Medical Officer of Health (M'Gonigle),[8] as discussed below.

Most of the research in nutrition supported by the MRC was on vitamins and other micronutrients. This work has been critically assessed by Celia Petts.[9] Work by Chick and others on the importance of total food intake, supported by the

MRC, was ignored in the advice the MRC gave to the Ministry of Health in the 1930s.[10]

The MRC in its concern with nutrition included under this heading caries and other dental problems, particularly in children.

In its early statements (1918–1919) it emphasised that "… from the beginning of their work the MRC have had in view the early investigation of a widespread inquiry into the chief factors contributing to infant mortality, both antenatal and postnatal. Much of the present high mortality is obviously due to general preventable causes like maternal ignorance, urbanisation and improper housing, and also imperfect feeding. But while available knowledge is already far ahead of effective administrative action in these respects, there are many factors contributing to a high infant death-rate which are at present quite imperfectly understood. It is clear, moreover, that our knowledge of the causes of many still births and premature births is lacking chiefly for the want of organised scientific work."[4] This presaged a series of statistical studies of child health, particularly in Scotland – but it cannot be said to have been in the forefront of the MRC's research efforts.

Landsborough Thompson[4] describes a series of investigations supported and initiated by the MRC in the period up to 1939, including important work on obstetrics and maternal infections.

The MRC was very concerned at the lack of significant research in pathology and bacteriology. This was noted in its report in 1923–24 in which it commented on the compulsion of university departments of pathology and bacteriology to earn money by "engaging largely in routine examinations for public health authorities and medical practitioners, while the pathologists of the teaching hospitals had to earn much of their living in private practice". Only after World War II was the Public Health Laboratory Service created to relieve hospital and university laboratories of this burden. The emergency PHLS was created in 1941 under Dr Scott, who was killed in an accident shortly after appointment and was succeeded by Dr GS Wilson. The PHLS was at first under the umbrella of the MRC and only transferred to the NHS in 1958. From the start it had a strong research element, particularly in bacteriology and infectious disease.[11]

Apart from its support for statistical analyses of the incidence of a variety of infections, particularly tuberculosis, the MRC supported for many years an experimental approach to the subject of infection, initiated by Professor WWC Topley and his co-workers, including Professor Major Greenwood, first in Manchester and later at the London School of Hygiene. This consisted of experiments on a community of mice, maintained under controlled conditions. The investigations were to try to assess the effect of individual factors such as density, carriers and proportion of susceptibles on the spread of an epidemic. It is unfortunate that, in spite of considerable expenditure of time and effort, little of practical use resulted from this major MRC investment .

At this time the Council also supported a series of studies on diphtheria, scarlet fever and measles, in boarding schools and naval establishments. Work was also supported on virology, in particular the isolation of the influenza virus.

The history of the involvement of the MRC in tuberculosis research between the wars is dealt with in detail by Linda Bryden.[5] She comments that, despite the fact that concern with tuberculosis before 1914 was the main reason for the foundation of the MRC, by 1919 and later, "little real interest was shown by the Medical Research Council in this disease". This lack of interest was bolstered by the lack of pressure from the medical establishment until the appointment of Dr D'Arcy Hart at University College Hospital in the late 1930s. Perhaps the best illustration was the absence of any involvement or concern in the development of a vaccine – this attitude may have been at least partially justified after the disaster in Lübeck in 1929–30 when 72 out of 251 vaccinated children died of tuberculosis as a result of a contaminated batch of BCG.[10]

Research into infectious disease is an area where co-operation between various authorities is required if appropriate and innovative research designed to prevent such disease is to be planned. Between the wars such co-operation was sadly missing, as recounted by Bryden. This appears to have been partly the result of a clash of personalities between Sir Walter Fletcher, First Secretary of the MRC and Sir George Newman, Chief Medical Officer. But, in retrospect, the lack of interest by scientists involved in existing laboratory research as well as the inability of those in the field and in responsible administrative positions to influence politically determined conservative policies in the face of a depression could also be held to blame. Nonetheless the MRC did support a variety of infectious disease studies as noted above.

The attitude, funding and behaviour of the MRC changed somewhat after World War II. The emphasis on pure research remained but the organisation became more concerned with clinical medicine than before. Undoubtedly, the MRC had fostered a scientific approach to clinical medicine before 1939. The best example of this is the support of Sir Thomas Lewis at University College, the progenitor of many outstanding experimental scientific clinicians, such as Sir George Pickering, Edward Sharpey Schaefer and many others. In the early period, the leadership of the MRC had been in the hands of enlightened basic scientists, primarily physiologists. (Fletcher, Mellanby). It is possible that this change in attitude was linked to the arrival of Harold (later Sir Harold) Himsworth, an eminent member of Sir Thomas Lewis's Department at University College Hospital. Closer links also began to be developed with the Ministry of Health, although a degree of friction between the two persisted.

The behaviour of the MRC may also have been linked to the experience of senior clinicians and other scientists during the war, where the utility of epidemiology and public health in general was seen as crucial to the maintenance of health, not only of the armed forces but also of the general population. This change in attitude has been described[2] and will be dealt with later. The practical result was the creation of a number of MRC units specifically concerned with EPHR: Social Medicine Research Unit (Prof J N Morris), Epidemiological Research Unit, South Wales (Prof AL Cochrane), Pneumoconiosis Research Unit (Prof CM Fletcher and later Dr J Gilson[6]), Air Pollution Research Unit (Prof P Lawther), Social Psychiatry Research Unit (Prof J Wing), Unit for Research on the Epidemiology of Mental Illness (Prof GM Carstairs succeeded by Prof N Kessel, succeeded by Prof N Kreitman) and Unit for Obstetrics and Sociology (Sir Dugald Baird succeeded by Prof R Illsley). Other relevant units established were concerned with population genetics and addictions. The MRC also developed a programme of research in epidemiology, advised by a number of specific disease committees – for example, on chronic bronchitis, and later a "general epidemiology committee".

Perhaps the best examples of how the MRC developed and supported important work in the early period after the war was the work on treatment of tuberculosis, leading to the landmark study using a randomised control trial, the design of which was supervised by Bradford Hill. Equally significant was the work on cigarette smoking and cancer of the lung under the direction of Bradford Hill in collaboration with Richard Doll. The MRC did not only foster EPHR, but also provided training fellowships for individuals wishing to develop their expertise in EPHR, and international research training fellowships in collaboration with the US Public Health Service (USPHS).

The MRC did not confine itself to supporting research – it also attempted to influence public policy, even in areas of extreme political sensitivity, as a result of the findings of research it supported. Thus it was one of the first public bodies to pronounce on the dangers of smoking in 1957.

It is not the purpose of this book to describe, in detail, the research in EPHR supported by any individual body. It is sufficient to record that the MRC was generous in its support in the period up to about 1970.

At this time, pressures on resources began to increase. This was caused by the increased possibilities of undertaking research as a result of the development of scientific methods and partly by the need to restrict expenditures for general economic reasons. The MRC, once again, began a slow general retreat from the investigation of applied problems, back to concentrating on basic research.

During this period, the government of the day began to question the value of and need for scientific research. As a result it established an enquiry under Lord Rothschild whose report recommended that a system of identifying customer-contractor principles should be introduced. These "principles" in essence were that Government departments should identify what research was required to determine and evaluate their policies and that they should then commission the necessary research. This, of course, is an easy principle to apply in applied engineering research, for example, but far more difficult in basic biomedical research, or even in the more applied public health research field.

Controversially, the Medical Research Council was enjoined to devote a proportion of its budget to what became known as "Rothschild" research. The membership of the Council was supplemented by nominees of the Department of Health, and some of the MRC work was labelled appropriately. Apart from the difficulties experienced by the MRC and researchers in applying these principles, the Department of Health had difficulties in formulating appropriate, researchable "questions". This led to a great deal of turmoil in the research world which is cogently described in various Nuffield Provincial Hospitals Trust and other publications.[12–15]

By 1984, the system settled down; the compromises reached have been described and are not relevant here. The policy of the MRC towards EPHR has now become very sympathetic and the organisation has developed a specific strategic role in promoting it. In order to fulfil this role it not only supports specific research in developing methodology and high priority areas of research, but also has taken a major role in training for public health research, through both junior and senior research fellowships. The MRC's current portfolio for research, its priority areas and the description of its role are well described in the MRC reports. In 1981 the MRC decided that applications for support in health services research (HSR) should be fed into the existing Boards and Grants machinery but that in addition an HSR panel should be set up to advise the Boards and Council. This was purely an advisory body.

In 1986 it was renamed the HSR Committee and in 1991 became the HSR and Public Health Research Board. In 1999 the MRC published a strategic review of the future support for epidemiology. This review highlighted important future trends and priorities for funding as well as training, recruitment and career problems which the MRC could help to tackle.

Ministry of Health
1919–1939
The Ministry at this time had no formal research funding mechanisms. Although individual projects of high priority were funded, these were ad hoc in nature and concerned specific one-off problems. Some "operational" research was done by ministry staff – for example, studies of morbidity and mortality by the Ministry's Regional Medical officers in areas of high unemployment during the early 1930s. This work cannot be considered as true research and was roundly criticised because it investigated problems of political concern and could, therefore, be interpreted as upholding governmental policies rather than evaluating them critically. As was shown by Lewis Fanning,[16] it was unlikely to show an acute effect, as the areas investigated had a long history of deprivation. Research required by the Ministry was undertaken through co-ordinating mechanisms with the MRC and, as has already been discussed, often led to disagreements between the two bodies.

1945–1969

The post-war period was dominated by the introduction of the National Health Service[17] which absorbed all Ministerial energies. The only "research" studies which the Ministry was really interested in were surveys of public opinion regarding the NHS in terms of use of the new service, and economic questions on its costs which culminated in the Guillebaud Inquiry.[18] This latter commissioned some extremely important and innovative research on the costs of the NHS by Professor Richard Titmuss and his research assistant Brian Abel-Smith. But apart from these rare exceptions, little interest was demonstrated.

By the mid 1960s the need for EPHR became more manifest. Although the MRC did provide support in this field, its major concerns were with basic medical research, and although it supported a number of research units, the need was much greater and was not met. A very small amount of money (£3000) was available through the medical division of the Ministry, largely because of the foresight of a principal, John Cornish, who had served in operational research in the Navy during the war. The inadequacies of this were, however, apparent and as a result the Ministry began to develop its own funding mechanisms. It was fortunate in having Dr RHL Cohen as Deputy Chief Medical Officer, who had previously been Third Secretary of the MRC and who clearly understood the need for this type of research. The subsequent development of the research and development division, and the units and programmes it supported, have been well described.[12,13]

Department of Health and Social Security
1970–1998

There was some progress in the research supported by the new Department of Health and Social Security. Difficulties, however, began to occur at the beginning of the 1980s, as described by Kember and Macpherson.[19]

The decline in both quality and quantity of medical research came to public notice and led to an external review by a sub-committee of the House of Lords in 1987–8.[20] The enquiry was exhaustive and its opinion began by stating (3.1), "the committee could not fail to be impressed, from the tone of all the evidence received, by the atmosphere of despondency that reflected the low morale of those engaged in medical research. It is not only that funding is so inadequate that good research proposals are not supported, it is not only that career prospects in research are often dismal, it is not only that patient care frequently inhibits research activity, important as all these factors are. The overriding cause of the collapse of morale is the impression, right or wrong, that neither the NHS nor the DHSS demonstrates any awareness of the importance of research nor is prepared to devote time, effort and resources to promote it, save only when either an immediate saving of money is in prospect or when public concern, as in the case of AIDS, forces its hand.

"Either the Government considers that medical research does not matter or else it has simply failed to convey to the medical community and the public the fact that it thinks medical research does matter."

The committee was particularly concerned with difficulties of applied research or, as they called it, public health and operational research. It regarded the mechanisms established by the Department of Health as inadequate, both in asking those dealing with the development of health policy to consider what research was required and in applying research findings. It argued that EPHR had been inadequately supported in the UK and that the amount and organisation of such research needed reform.

Although the committee argued for the establishment of an independent National Health Research Authority, the Government, in its response to the report, declined to establish such an authority. Instead they created a Research Directorate with a Director of Permanent Secretary status as its head and with a seat on the NHS Management Executive.

The programme of work and its role over the first decade are described by Peckham in his Rock Carling Lecture.[21] After initial optimism by public health researchers, disillusion quickly set in. There was a great difference between the recommendations of the House of Lords for the development of EPHR and the research developed by the new directorate whose main aim became the promotion of clinical and health services research.[19] Much of the available resource was directed not to new research but to relabelling existing or old work.

With the change of government in 1997, there are signs that the Directorate, under its third Director, is now beginning to fulfil the role originally envisaged.

Public Health Laboratory Service (PHLS)

The PHLS was created during World War II and was under the MRC until 1958. Its history and work have been well described, most recently, by Sir Robert Williams, a former Director.[11] The PHLS has always been concerned with the epidemiology of infectious disease. At the beginning there was an Epidemiological Research Laboratory, which was incorporated into the present Communicable Disease Surveillance Centre. These have always undertaken appropriate research internally and some of the original, important work undertaken, for example, in vaccine evaluation and control (and spread) of infection have already been discussed.

Public Health Departments, Local Authorities, Health Authorities

1919–1939

Public Health Departments during this time were not much concerned with either the support or the conduct of research. The major and most significant exception to this was in Stockton-On-Tees where Dr M'Gonigle undertook his very important work, first on the effect of housing on health and later on the impact of poverty on diet. It is noteworthy that in later years his work was supported by the MRC.[8]

Public Health Departments were also involved in trials of prevention including evaluation of sera, spread of infection, outbreak investigation and developing methods of prevention as well as delivery of public health services.

1945–1974

After the inception of the NHS, the role of EPHR in local authorities and health authorities was mainly in the provision of facilities and manpower to do research rather than to initiate studies. Examples were in the provision of facilities for testing immunising agents, evaluation of domiciliary midwifery, and health centres. In some instances there was even more involvement: in studies of respiratory disease in school children in four areas of Kent to determine the effect of air pollution on health, for example, the County Council not only included the necessary investigations in the work of its medical officers and school nurses but also trained them to provide reliable results.[22] This informal approach of including research in the "normal" work of the service was common in all parts of medical research in the UK at that time.

Health Authorities (Hospital Management Committee (HMC), Regional Hospital Board (RHB), Area Health Authority (AHA), District Health Authority (DHA), Regional Health Authority (RHA)) *1974–1998*

As noted above, the interest of the NHS in EPHR was not great. Funds for research were available under a scheme known as "locally organised research" and administered at the regional level. The sums available were very small, and were mostly spent on straight clinical research. Epidemiological research was helped in an informal, non-remunerated manner by staff keeping special research records, particularly in research enquiries and undertaking additional pathological or other tests for research.

With the inclusion of public health within the NHS structure, EPHR continued to be supported in the same way as in the past. It was not until the Directorate of Research was created at the Department of Health, after the House of Lords Inquiry, that each Region also acquired a Director of Research. The disappointing result of this has been described above.

Charitable Foundations

The role of charitable foundations in the support of EPHR has been critical throughout this century. The London School of Hygiene was created as a result of a grant by the Rockefeller Foundation.[23] Before World War II, the Carnegie Foundation was also responsible for some of the crucial work demonstrating the effect of adequate nutrition in school children. British foundations played only minor roles in support of EPHR before 1939.

After 1945, the Nuffield Provincial Hospitals Trust played a crucial role in the development and strengthening of EPHR, well described by McLachlan.[24] Not only did they provide funds for the foundation of the Chairs in Social Medicine in Oxford and Birmingham, but they have continued uninterruptedly to promote EPHR for 50 years. The sums of money available for disbursement by the Trust have never been great (now about £1 million per annum) but they have used their funds imaginatively as a catalyst and probe to foster EPHR.

The Nuffield Foundation has also fostered some work, for example, on cross-infection in hospitals, but has left the field open to the Trust.

Since 1948, the King's Fund, founded in 1897 for the support of London Hospitals, has also played a small role in the support of EPHR, in particular by concentrating on health/medical services.

Other foundations, such as the Wolfson, have also supported EPHR. The wealthiest of all foundations since 1987, the Wellcome, has provided significant support for training in epidemiology and infectious disease research, with a particular emphasis on the needs of developing countries.

Most of the voluntary hospitals had "endowment" funds from voluntary contributions. They were able to retain these, after the hospitals were nationalised in 1948, for expenditure on research. Although the funds available in most were trivial, there were some in teaching hospitals such as St Bartholomews' and St Thomas's which, in the 1970s and later, had at least £5 million available for research annually. This could be used for EPHR, although most of the money was spent on clinical research.

Voluntary Bodies

Important players in funding EPHR have always been single-disease charities. These are now grouped together under the heading "Association of Medical Research Charities". They have a long history. The National Association for Tuberculosis, for example, was founded over 100 years ago. Over this period it has changed its name several times, first to Tuberculosis and Chest Disease, then to Chest and Heart, then to Chest Heart and Stroke and in 1993 to The Stroke Association. During this time the Association has funded and promoted EPHR under its various titles.

The big players now provide funds for research on cancer (Imperial Cancer Research Fund (ICRF), Cancer Research Campaign, both now amalgamated to form Cancer Research UK) and heart disease (British Heart Foundation). These large charities each support relatively short-term research projects, some of which include EPHR questions. They also support professorial appointments, longer term research programmes and units, as well as training in research. Some of this support, although it is not possible to quantify the proportion, is directed towards EPHR. Most of the grants are for research considered relevant to individual patient care, including clinical, basic, behavioural and social, but a significant proportion is spent on EPHR. The Stroke Association, for example, spends about one-third of a total research expenditure of about £2 million per annum on EPHR.

Conclusion

Before 1939, funds for EPHR were scanty. Neither the universities, Medical Research Council, government, nor other administrative bodies viewed expenditure on EPHR as a priority at a time of great poverty and unemployment. By contrast, charitable bodies, particularly some in America, such as the Rockefeller and Carnegie foundations, were generous in supporting institutions for EPHR and programmes intended to alleviate health problems resulting from current economic conditions.

Between 1945 and 1969 the Medical Research Council, in particular, devoted increasing attention to EPHR, and the universities also began to develop an interest. During this period, an English charitable foundation, the Nuffield Provincial Hospitals Trust (NPHT), was also prominent in supporting and encouraging research in this field.

Since 1970 there has been marked although sporadic development in the provision of resources and greater interest in EPHR from many sources and, in particular, from the universities and the Department of Health. Foundations, voluntary bodies and the MRC have maintained their interest and funding.

APPENDIX

Examples of Development of Academic Departments in the United Kingdom

Details from each academic department in England, Scotland, Wales and Northern Ireland have been received. The examples given have been chosen to illustrate the development of the subject.

Glasgow

The Department was founded in 1923 with the endowment of a Chair in Public Health. In 1932 the name was changed to the Institute of Hygiene, in 1965 to Epidemiology and Preventive Medicine and in 1989 to Public Health. JR Currie was Professor from 1923 to 1940. There was an additional assistant lecturer between 1924 and 1928, with a second appointment in 1928 and a third in 1931. J McIntosh was Professor from 1940 to 1943 and had 10 lecturers. He was succeeded by T Ferguson from 1944 to 1963 and he had initially three lecturers, increasing to six senior lecturers. In 1964 T Anderson became Professor, and the Department increased to eight or nine other staff. GT Stewart was professor from 1972 to 1983 with six or seven other staff. AJ Hedley succeeded him till 1989, to be followed by J McEwen. Staffing at this time rose to nine and in 1990 to 13, two being part-time appointments.

Belfast

The Department of Public Health was founded in 1896. WJ Wilson was professor in 1925 with one assistant. By 1940 he had three assistants. Wilson was succeeded in 1945 by AC Stevenson who by 1952 had five assistants. The Department changed its name at this time to Social and Preventive Medicine. John Pemberton succeeded to the Chair in 1958; he retired in 1976 and was succeeded by Harold Ellwood who was then succeeded by Alan Evans. The number of full-time additional staff was never less than five, and the Department published more than 1200 original papers between 1947 and 1998.

Manchester

The Department was founded in 1891 when A Sheridan Delépine was appointed as Professor of Public Health and Bacteriology. Other Professors were HB Maitland (1927–62), A Topping (1947–50), CF Brockington (1951–64), EA Smith (1967–1979), IM Leck (1979–1991), and SDB Donnan (1990–1997). There were always two or more lecturers/senior lecturers.

Newcastle

In 1873 Henry Amstrong was appointed Medical Officer of Health (MOH) in Newcastle and became Lecturer (later Professor) in Public Health in 1874. He was succeeded by TE Hill (1911–20) and H Kerr (1920–33), both Medical Officers of Health, and they were succeeded by J Charles (1933–44), McCracken (1945–46), WS Walton (1947–56) and then RCM Pearson until 1964. The first pure university appointment was J Walker (1964–86). Raj Bhopal was Senior Lecturer, and then Professor (1988–98). The first additional university lectureship was created in 1977 when D Foster was appointed Senior Lecturer, between 1964 and 1986. The department was a joint general practice and public health one, with Dr Walker's main interest being in the former.

Wales

The Mansel Talbot Chair was endowed in 1918, the first full-time Chair in epidemiology and public health. The first holder was EL Collins and there were four additional lecturers. Picken succeeded to the Chair in 1933, and by F Grundy in 1948. By 1951 there were six additional university appointments. CR Lowe was Professor from 1962–88, C Roberts 1988–1997 and SR Palmer since 1997.

The London / St Bartholomew's Hospital Medical College (University of London)

Eva Alberman was appointed Professor of Clinical Epidemiology in 1979. Bart's formally opened a Department in 1983 when NJ Wald was appointed as Head. The college emphasises its interest by noting that there was a lecturer from 1950–58 in public health, and a variety of eminent individuals, such as Sir George Newman, who gave lectures in earlier years.

St Thomas' Hospital Medical School (University of London)

Sir John Simon, Medical Officer of Health to the city of London (1848–1855) and subsequently the first Chief Medical Officer to the Local Government Board, predecessor of the Ministry of Health (1856–1876), was also a teacher at St Thomas' in surgery. He was very concerned that future doctors should be taught public health. As a result St Thomas' appointed the first British full-time lecturer in epidemiology and public health in 1855 (W Greenhow, 1855–1861). After his departure to a Chair at the Middlesex Hospital, no further academic appointment was made until 1961 when Walter Holland was appointed Senior Lecturer in Social Medicine within the Medical Unit charged with developing teaching and research in epidemiology. This was the first full-time appointment in any London Medical School for more than 100 years. The post became "independent" in 1964, and WWH was made Reader and then later Professor in 1968. He retired in 1994 and was succeeded by P Burney. From 1968 it housed a Social Medicine and Health Services Research Unit with about 30 academic staff.

REFERENCES

1 Pemberton J. (1998) Social medicine comes on the scene in the United Kingdom. 1936–1960. *Journal of Public Health Medicine*, 20: 149–163.

2 Holland WW. (1994) Changing names. *Scandinavian Journal of Social Medicine*, 22: 1–6.

3 Clarke M, Kurinczuk JJ. (1992) Health Services Research: a case of need or special pleading. *British Medical Journal*, 304: 1675–1676.

4 Landsborough Thompson A. (1975) *Half a Century of Medical Research*. Vols I and II. London: HMSO.

5 Austoker J, Bryden L, (Eds). (1989) *Historical Perspectives on the Role of the MRC*. Oxford: Oxford University Press.

6 Cotes JE. (2000) Medical Research Council Pneumoconiosis Research Unit 1945–1985: a short history and tribute. *Occupational Medicine*, 50: 440–449.

7 Orr JB. (1936) *Food, Health and Income*. London: Macmillan.

8 M'Gonigle GCM, Kirby J. (1936) *Poverty and Public Health*. London: Victor Gollancz.

9 Petts C. (1989) Nutrition research. In: *Historical Perspectives on the Role of the MRC*. Oxford: Oxford University Press, pp 83–108.

10 Report (1935) Die Säuglingstuberkulose in Lübeck. *Arbeiten aus dem Reichsgesundheitsamt*, 69: 1.

11 Williams REO. (1985) *Microbiology for the Public Health. The Evolution of the Public Health Laboratory Service 1939–1980*. London: Public Health Laboratory Service.

12 McLachlan G (Ed). (1971) *Portfolio for Health. The Role and Programme of the DHSS in Health Services Research*. London: Nuffield Provincial Hospitals Trust/ Oxford University Press.

13 McLachlan G (Ed). (1973) *Portfolio for Health 2. The Developing Programme of the DHSS in Health Services Research.* London: Nuffield Provincial Hospitals Trust/ Oxford University Press.

14 McLachlan G (Ed). (1978) *Five Years After. A Review of Health Care Research Management.* London: Nuffield Provincial Hospitals Trust/Oxford University Press.

15 Kogan M, Henkel M. (1983) *Government and Research. The Rothschild Experiment in a Government Department.* London: Heinemann Educational.

16 Lewis Fanning E. (1937) A study of the trend of mortality rates in urban communities of England and Wales with specific reference to depressed areas. *Lancet,* 1: 865–867.

17 Holland WW, Stewart S. (1998) *Public Health: The Vision and the Challenge.* London: Nuffield Trust.

18 *Report of the Committee of Inquiry into the Cost of the National Health Service* (the Guillebaud Report). (1956) London: HMSO, Cmnd 9663.

19 Kember T, Macpherson G. (1994) *The NHS – a Kaleidoscope of Care – Conflicts of Service and Business Values.* London: Nuffield Provincial Hospitals Trust.

20 Select Committee on Science and Technology. (1988) Priorities in Medical Research. London: HMSO, HL Paper 54-I.

21 Peckham M. (2000) *A Model for Health.* London: Nuffield Trust.

22 Holland WW, Halil T, Bennett AE, Elliott A. (1969) Factors influencing the onset of chronic respiratory disease. *British Medical Journal,* 2: 205.

23 Fee E, Acheson RM (Eds). (1991) *A History of Education in Public Health.* Oxford: Oxford University Press.

24 McLachlan G. (1992) *A History of the Nuffield Provincial Hospitals Trust 1940–1990.* London: Nuffield Provincial Hospitals Trust.

THE UNITED STATES

The support of EPHR has been different in the United States, both in method and in scale. The major differences are a result of the presence of a number of Schools of Public Health within universities and a national organisation, the US Public Health Service (USPHS), with a long tradition of concern with both the investigation of public health questions and the implementation of control measures. Furthermore, charitable foundations have played a major role both in investment in institutions and in supporting research.

Universities

1919–1939

In contrast to the UK, physicians active in public health were often considered the elite of their profession – examples are Stephen Smith, a founder of the American Public Health Association, Hermann Briggs, the great public health administrator of New York State, who also maintained a highly successful private medical practice, and William Henry Welch, the Dean of John Hopkins School of Medicine.[1]

Viseltear, in Fee and Acheson, describes the background to the development of Schools of Public Health in some detail.[1] The need for a scientific basis of education in public health was recognised and a variety of courses developed for doctors, engineers and others. By 1919, recognised Schools with well-developed courses were present in Harvard, Yale, Michigan, Columbia, Pennsylvania and Johns Hopkins Universities.

Of these, Johns Hopkins, supported by a Rockefeller endowment, served as a pattern for the development of the modern School of Public Health. Hopkins and Harvard were clearly oriented to research and had close links to their medical schools. By 1936, in addition to these six schools, four other universities, California at Berkeley, Minnesota, Wayne State in Detroit and the Massachusetts Institute of Technology offered courses in public health and were engaged in some form of research. The Rockefeller Foundation had emphasised the need for Schools of Public Health to be concerned with scientific rather than social research and this is one of the reasons they chose Johns Hopkins for their benefaction in view of the excellent scientific status of its medical school.

Although most of the students (63%) at Johns Hopkins were medical graduates, this was not necessarily the case at other Schools of Public Health – Michigan, for example, only had 25% medical graduates.[2]

The teaching and research in medical schools of epidemiology and public health was not well supported. The subject was usually labelled "preventive medicine" and as in the UK there were few, if any, medical schools, other than those associated with Schools of Public Health, that had very active departments. These were usually linked to bacteriology (microbiology) and the most eminent researchers were involved in studying infectious diseases, for example, polio by Paul at Yale.

As Fee[3] relates, the hope that public health and medicine would consummate a fruitful marriage was not realised and Nelson[4] notes the serious tensions between the two subjects and the attractions of acute medicine for the medical student. This was further exacerbated by the concept that those in public health were proponents of national health insurance (socialised medicine), opposed by most active clinicians.[5] The increase in the ability of public health to investigate and control infectious disease was also a source of friction with private practitioners.[6]

The hope that medical students would increasingly be attracted to public health, partly because of increased federal funding in response to the Depression and the increase in state expenditures on public health, was not realised. The growing domination of hospital (institutional) medicine with increasing medical knowledge dependent on scientific knowledge and technology was a powerful attraction to medical students and graduates. Thus, as in the UK between 1945 and 1969, few medical graduates were attracted to public health with its relatively low incomes as compared to private practice, its political pressures and its comparative lack of individual autonomy.

1946–1969
Of major importance in the development of academic organisations in the post-war decades was a new congressional interest in medical research.[7] Congress's support of research diverted interest from comprehensive federal health care provision until 1965 when the Medicare – Medicaid Legislation was introduced.

As in the UK, there was great expansion in universities and research funding in the USA after World War II. In the late 1940s there were seven major Schools of

Public Health: John Hopkins, Harvard, Michigan, North Carolina, Columbia, California and Minnesota. About one-third of the students were medical graduates, the remainder were mainly sanitary engineers, health educators and nurses. About 50% of the medical graduates and two-thirds of the engineers were from abroad. By 1947 a further two schools were accredited, Vanderbilt and Yale, although several other universities provided training in public health (for example, Chicago, Indiana, Massachusetts Institute of Technology, New York University, Oregon, Pennsylvania, Rutgers, St Louis, Syracuse, Washington, Wayne and Western Reserve). In 1948–49 Vanderbilt dropped from the list and Tulane was added, to be joined by Pittsburgh in 1950 and 1951, and Puerto Rico and UCLA in 1960–62.

The research output of the different schools was proportional to the size of the faculty, and it was thought that the faculty spent about 40% of their time on research. Of all the faculties active in research, 40% were based at John Hopkins and Harvard.[1]

The number of medical schools expanded to 113 after World War II. There was a great expansion in student enrolment, with a 50% increase between 1965 and 1975.[4]

There were a number of medical schools active in EPHR at this time, other than those with Schools of Public Health. A number, such as Pennsylvania, Rutgers, St Louis, Syracuse, Wayne and Western Reserve have already been referred to above as providing training in public health. But, in addition, medical schools at Rochester (NY), Duke (NC) Vermont (VT) and Birmingham (AL) in particular, were active in EPHR. Of particular note is that the University of California at Los Angeles (UCLA) had a very active department of preventive medicine which, toward the end of this period, developed into a separate School of Public Health but retained its administrative and educational link to the medical school.

The major emphasis, however, of research funding in universities at this time was in basic sciences and clinical medicine.

1970–1998
The link between local health departments and Schools of Public Health weakened as the schools became more dependent on federal funding. The latter

increased, not only because of greater interest in the types of research undertaken by Schools of Public Health, but also because of increased federal concern with poverty and the increasing need for medical care administrators to deal with new federal initiatives such as Medicare and Medicaid.

Between 1958 and 1973 the number of students in Schools of Public Health quadrupled.[1] The new students were attracted into the field not only because of the increase in student federal funding but also because of the widening of the scope of Schools of Public Health from their concern with infectious disease to consideration of international health, chronic disease, family planning and health administration. Seven new Schools were accredited between 1965 and 1972 – Hawaii, Loma Linda, Texas, Oklahoma, Washington, Massachusetts, Illinois – and five more between 1973 and 1989 at South Carolina, Alabama, Boston, San Diego State and South Florida.

The mix of students also changed; in 1988 about 22% were medical graduates and 8% nurses. The proportion of medical graduates varied from about 5% at Massachusetts to 46% at Harvard. The proportion of medical graduates from overseas remained unchanged, at about 50%.

The proportion of medical graduates at Schools of Public Health continued to fall; in 1998–1999 only about 15% were medical graduates, of whom 31% were foreign nationals (in contrast to 47% in 1988–1989). At the same time the total number of graduate students has risen from 2824 to 4720 between 1998 and 1999.

The acceptance that public health knowledge and its application are multi-disciplinary had been dominant in the USA since the beginning of the twentieth century. The Schools of Public Health created all demonstrated these principles, although the contribution of medically qualified practitioners was dominant at the start, as shown by the location of the premier school, Johns Hopkins, adjacent to the Hospital and Medical School. This emphasis has changed markedly over time – so that by the end of the twentieth century the great majority of both staff and students were not medically qualified.

While all Schools of Public Health are parts of universities, they remain very independent and there are wide variations among them in the type of research they do, their educational programmes and their student mix.

Federal Funding of EPHR

In the US, EPHR falls under the broad category of biomedical research. The US spends more money on biomedical research than any other country in the world but the proportion of that funding spent on EPHR is impossible to determine. It is unlikely, however, to be a large proportion.[8]

The actual amounts of money spent on different forms of research are difficult to disentangle from total funding, although Braun has made some attempt at this.[9] He shows that in all areas the US spends at least twice as much as the UK. The rise in research and development expenditure in the USA is illustrated by comparing 1980 and 1995.[10] Federal expenditure rose from $8865 million to $13442 million (at constant dollars), and this does not include federally funded research.

In 1891, the Hygienic Laboratory was organised by the Marine Hospital Service (later US Public Health Service) and became the focus for epidemiological research.[6] As has already been mentioned, it was the training ground of many future leaders of US public health research such as Rosenau, Wade Hampton Frost and Comstock. The Hygienic Laboratory did not limit itself to infectious disease but also tackled such problems as pellagra (at one time considered to be of bacterial origin).

Medical research grew in stature over the years. In 1930 an Act was passed creating the National Institutes of Health (NIH). Initially, this only meant a change in name of the Hygienic Laboratory. As Fitzhugh-Mullen[11] recounts, however, Cumming, Parran and others envisioned greatly expanded facilities in the future – impeded only by the lack of funds at this time as a result of the Depression. In 1935 Mr and Mrs Luke Wilson offered their estate in suburban Bethesda to the government as the new site for the NIH.

The NIH had gradually started to shift its research from infectious to non-infectious disease. The National Cancer Institute (NCI) had inaugurated the categorical approach to NIH research where funds and facilities were devoted to a particular group of diseases. The legislation also provided a new approach, an extramural grant programme in support of cancer researchers at other institutions than the NIH.

Research in non-infectious disease epidemiology in the UK developed primarily as an academic discipline. This was quite different from the situation in the USA, where epidemiological research had developed primarily as a function of federal, state, and local health departments.[12]

After World War II there was further expansion in federal epidemiology. The Communicable Disease Center was founded in 1946 by conversion of the wartime Office of Malaria Control in War Areas; it is now the Center for Disease Control, Atlanta. It is concerned with a variety of infectious and non-infectious diseases.

The Public Health Service (PHS) Act of 1944 broadened the commissioned corps, authorising the commissioning of nurses, scientists, dieticians, physical therapists and sanitarians. It also specified a new organisation for the PHS: the office of the Surgeon General and three "bureaux" – State Services, Medical Services and the NIH. This lasted for the next 20 years.

This account is not intended to chronicle all the administrative changes which have occurred in the PHS and NIH over the years. It is, however, worth recording some of the salient events which have influenced the direction of research policies and their application in practice.

The transfer of all native Indian health programmes to the PHS in 1955 with associated funding for improvement of health and environmental facilities was associated, by 1960, with a major reduction of infant mortality and tuberculosis. The programmes in these two areas were greatly influenced by the previous research done by the PHS.

The CDC established the Epidemic Intelligence Service (EIS) in 1951 under Dr Alexander Langmuir. He applied the training he had received at Johns Hopkins under Wade Hampton Frost to developing a national (and later international) capacity to investigate outbreaks of disease and institute proper methods of surveillance and control.

Fee and Brown[13] have suggested that this was done partly to prepare for the possibility of biological warfare, a great fear at the time of the Korean War. They further suggest that this channelled federal energies on the surveillance of infectious disease and delayed concern with development of programmes in chronic disease until the 1960s and 1970s.

Perhaps one of the most noteworthy examples of the application of research to health policy was the establishment by Surgeon General, Luther Terry, in 1962, of an Advisory Committee on Smoking and Health. The publication of their report in 1964 was a major landmark of the recognition by a major government of the health risks of tobacco.[14]

The variety, scope and size of research funding sources and institutions involved in EPHR in the USA is both large and bewildering. It is illustrated and described by Detels and colleagues.[8] The NIH comprises 21 separate agencies such as the National Cancer Institute, National Heart, Lung, and Blood Institute, National Institute for the Environmental Sciences and so on. There is no single focus for public health research, although each institute usually has a branch devoted to epidemiology and one to statistics. When NIH first started, most of its research was conducted intramurally and powers to fund extramural research were only given in 1937. The balance between intra- and extramural research has gradually shifted. In the early years most research was intramural; now most is extramural and the institutes serve essentially as administrative agents.

Most research funds from NIH are project grants in response to application from individual investigators. These are assessed by the usual methods of peer review. Each institute also has a council, which sets priorities for its field of interest in the hope that this will promote research in the areas chosen. In addition these councils may contract for specific, priority areas of research by inviting bids (requests for proposals – RFPs). Institutes may also promote research in specific areas of interest by issuing requests for applications (RFAs), which alert researchers that funds have been set aside for research in these areas and that proposals in these areas may receive priority funding. The setting of priorities for research may also come from the Office of the Director of NIH or from congressional mandates implemented through special provision of funds to NIH to research in designated specific areas. Examples of the latter were the emphasis on heart disease and stroke in the late 1960s and on cancer some years later.

The Center for Disease Control and Prevention (CDC) is the federal agency responsible for disease control in the United States. It does undertake appropriate epidemiological research to fulfil its primary function of disease surveillance and control. Although most research is done in-house, some is contracted to researchers in universities and particularly in Schools of Public Health.

The Environmental Protection Agency (EPA) has the responsibility for protecting the US public from environmental hazards. It conducts both intramural and extramural research, the latter through a contract and grants mechanism. This is similar to the procedures of the NIH. Its predecessor agency, the Division of Air Pollution, was created largely as a result of the disastrous air pollution incident in Donora, Pennsylvannia, in 1948.

The agency for Health Care Policy Research and the Health Care Financing Corporation are the major federal agencies involved in funding health services research. Most of the research is funded extramurally using similar mechanisms to NIH.

There are, in addition, several other federal agencies funding research relevant to public health – for example, the Federal Drugs Administration (FDA). All use similar mechanisms to those developed by NIH.

It can thus be seen that there are many sources of money for public health research – with little coordination between them. The amount of money available for health research from federal sources has increased steadily over the years – it more than doubled between 1983 and 1993.

State and Local Level Support

A few States and Counties provide support for EPHR. Examples at State level are California and New York. The former, for example, supports work on environmental hazards such as air pollution. At more local level, New York City and Los Angeles County have been prominent in the support of public health research – the former particularly in the control of diseases such as tuberculosis and in health services, the latter in environmental matters.

Private or Charitable Funding

Private foundations have played and continue to play a very major role in the funding of public health research. Even before the major contributions of the Rockefeller Foundation to the founding of the Johns Hopkins School of Hygiene, both this Foundation and the Carnegie Foundation had been involved in the support of EPHR.

The policies and role of these charities is well described by Brown[15] and Duffy.[16] It is interesting to speculate why, in the period between 1919 and 1939,

Americans were so willing to spend very large amounts of money on public health research, education and also practice. It is true that an enormous amount of wealth had been created in the United States toward the end of the nineteenth and beginning of the twentieth century and continued to accrue in the latter. It is difficult to make quantitative comparisons, but the amount of wealth created in the US as a result of the industrial expansion after the end of the Civil War was far greater than that created by the industrial revolution in the UK at the beginning of the nineteenth century. It is likely that individual wealth in the UK was similar to that of the US, but in the former it was "old", in the latter "new", money.

There are fundamental differences in the attitudes of the individuals who created this wealth between the US and UK. In the US, philanthropy was considered to be for the rehabilitation of the poor. Carnegie,[15] one of the first of the large donors, considered that "legacies undermine the moral integrity of the recipients" and believed that wealth should be thought of as a "trust fund" for society as a whole. Rockefeller and Gates, who presided over the disbursements of the Rockefeller Foundation, wished to use the wealth that the former had accumulated to shape the social and economic order. They considered that medicine was non-political and were adamant that their resources should not be used to help state enterprises – thus until the 1930s, Rockefeller money was only disbursed to private universities for the endowment of Schools of Medicine and Public Health.

WH Welch (of Johns Hopkins) was particularly influential in promoting the cause of medical research as a prime method for the use of science to improve life for the population. It has to be recognised, however, that some of the reasons may have been less altruistic – for example, the wish to head off socialism and provide counter-propaganda after the 1914 massacre of striking miners and their wives and children in a Ludlow, Colorado, mining company controlled by the Rockefellers.[15] Undoubtedly, this charitable expenditure, both in the past and now, is helped by US tax laws. Nonetheless the prime motivation appears to have been to create an appropriate environment for the development of professionals in public health and medicine at the beginning of the last century. In the nineteenth century American physicians were not held in high esteem.[16] It was not until the endowment of Johns Hopkins Medical School by the Rockefeller Foundation that scientific research in medicine really began to take off in the United States.

The enormous charitable support of health research in the United States over the years may also have had several other reasons. Many of the major donors at the beginning of the last century were self-made men who had experience of poverty. This may have influenced them in supporting activities that would alleviate some of the problems of poverty, and serve as a social investment. Both then and now, American society is far more individualistic than its British equivalent. American donations may be influenced by the belief that they enable individuals "to take charge", rather than the state. The most recent examples of this may be the development of "venture philanthropists".

This contrasts with UK private charitable foundations. There is no UK charitable foundation comparable to those in the US. Only the Nuffield Provincial Hospitals Trust (now the Nuffield Trust) specialises in the support of public health research, and its grants are minuscule in comparison. It is difficult to determine whether the same motivations encouraged Lord Nuffield in his charitable activities. He was also a self-made man, and he had no family to whom his wealth could be left.

The custom of support from large industrial foundations to sustain EPHR in the United States has persisted. As well as the Rockefeller and Carnegie Foundations, others have entered the field – Robert Wood Johnson, Commonwealth, Milbank, Kaiser Family Foundation and most recently Gates. The Robert Wood Johnson Foundation is probably one of the largest sources of funds for health services research in the United States.

Many of the foundations fund not only research but also the development of innovative programmes of disease control or health service development. In the 1920s, rural health programmes, particularly in the southern and western states, to control tuberculosis, were the result of joint work between the Rockefeller Foundation, Milbank Memorial Fund, the Kellogg Foundation and the Red Cross.[16]

In addition to these large foundations there are, as in the UK, a number of disease-specific voluntary associations such as the American Cancer Society, American Heart Association, American Foundation for Aids and, in the past, March of Dimes (polio). They have been in the forefront of supporting public health research in such matters as tobacco and diet. These disease-specific voluntary bodies also play a crucial role in advocacy to Congress for funds for research and control in their own field.

The commercial–industrial sector plays a significant role in the funding of public health research in the United States. The role of pharmaceutical companies in funding vaccine and treatment developments are similar in both countries. Industry in the United States, however, is more involved in funding research to define occupational/industrial hazards, and the evaluation of possible methods of organisation or equipment for the delivery of health services, such as screening.

Conclusion

The vast array of sources of funding, as well as of funds, in the United States as compared to the United Kingdom needs to be assessed critically.

Since the beginning of the last century, private philanthropy has been very active in the support of public health and its research capabilities. The involvement of federal resources in public health research has always had a defined structure – the US Public Health Service – and burgeoned after World War II through the development of NIH. The system of research support is, however, disorganised and lacks a unifying approach – probably because there is no unifying health system that can apply the findings. Between the two World Wars EPHR appeared to be driven by the concept that social deprivation should be alleviated. This was true of federal, state and private initiatives. Perhaps this can be attributed to the general effects of poverty in all parts of the USA as a result of the Depression. The effects of the latter in the UK were far more circumscribed and therefore did not lead to a universal remedial drive.

Since the end of World War II the dominance of "technical-scientific" research has been similar in the US and UK. The former, however, does not have a universal health system, so that there is no unifying structure which could help to identify the crucial areas for public health research. Thus US research is more "democratic" and "investigation" rather than "problem" driven.[6] The lack of structure also implies that the translation of research findings into health or health service policies is far more problematic.

APPENDIX
Schools of Public Health

1919–1936	Johns Hopkins
	Harvard
	Yale
	Michigan
	Columbia
	Pennsylvania
1936–1939	California at Berkeley
	Minnesota
	Wayne State
	Massachusetts Institute of Technology
1945	Johns Hopkins
	Harvard
	Michigan
	North Carolina
	Columbia
	California at Berkeley
	Minnesota
1946	Vanderbilt (ceased 1949)
	Yale
1949	Tulane
1950	Pittsburgh
1960–62	Puerto Rico
	California at Los Angeles (UCLA)
1965–1972	Hawaii
	Loma Linda
	Texas
	Oklahoma
	Washington
	Massachusetts
	Illinois

Schools of Public Health *(contd)*

1973–1989   South Carolina
                               Alabama
                               Boston
                               San Diego State
                               South Florida

**Medical Schools with Active Departments of
Public Health / Epidemiology**

Pre-1939   Pennsylvania
                               Rutgers
                               St Louis
                               Syracuse
                               Wayne
                               Western Reserve

After 1945 in addition   San Diego
                               Rochester
                               Cincinnati
                               Duke
                               Birmingham
                               UCLA
                               Vermont

REFERENCES

1 Fee E, Acheson RM (Eds). (1991) *A History of Education in Public Health*. Oxford: Oxford University Press.

2 Ludmerer KM. (1999) *Time to heal: American Medical Education From the Turn of the Century to the Era of Managed Care*. Oxford: Oxford University Press.

3 Fee E. (1989) Henry Sigerist: from the social production of disease to medical management and scientific socialism. *Milbank Quarterly*, 67: suppl 1, pp 127–150.

4 Nelson Russel A. (1974) Organisational relationships of school of public health with schools of medicine. In: *Schools of Public Health: Present and Future*. Bowers JZ, Purcell E (Eds). New York: Josiah Macy Jo Foundation, pp 11–14..

5 Duffy J. (1979) The American Medical Profession and public health – from support to ambivalence. *Bulletin of the History of Medicine*, 53: 1–22.

6 Cassedy JH. (1991) *Medicine in America*. Baltimore, MD: Johns Hopkins University Press.

7 Gemmell MK. (2001) Executive Director, Association of Schools of Public Health, personal communication.

8 Detels R, Holland WW, Tanaka H. (1996) Organisational status of basic and applied research in public health. In: *International Handbook of Public Health*. Hurrelman K, Laaser U (Eds). Westport, CT: Greenwood Press.

9 Braun D (1994) *Health Research and its Funding, Comparing France, England, Germany and the USA*. Bonn:Federal Ministry for Research and Technology.

10 Altbach PG, Beardahl RO, Gumport PJ, et al. (1999) *American Higher Education in the 21st Century: Social and Political Challenges*. Baltimore, MD: Johns Hopkins University Press.

11 Fitzhugh-Mullen M. (1989) *Plagues and Politics. The Story of the US Public Health Service*. New York: Basic Books.

12 Terris M. (1992) The society for epidemiologic research and the future of epidemiology. *American Journal of Epidemiology*, 136: 909–915.

13 Fee E, Brown TM. (2001) Pre-emptive biopreparedness: can we learn from history? *American Journal of Public Health*, 91: 721–726.

14 Report of the Public Health Service (1964) *Smoking and Health*. Washington DC: Public Health Service Publication No. 1103.

15 Brown ER. (1979) *Rockefeller Medicine Men, Medicine and Capitalism in America*. Berkeley, Los Angeles: University of California Press.

16 Duffy J. (1990) *The Sanitarians, A History of American Public Health*. Chicago: University of Illinois Press.

5. Trends in UK and US Society and Politics, 1919–1998

In this chapter, the main climate and concerns of society and politics in both the United Kingdom and the United States are discussed over three time periods: 1919–1939, 1945–1979 and 1980–1999, to provide a background against which EPHR was developing. The governments of the UK and the Presidents of the US are listed in appendices 1 and 2 at the end of the chapter.

THE UNITED KINGDOM 1919–1939
In spite of winning World War I, Britain emerged as a damaged society. About one million British men were killed and many more were injured. Britain had entered the war with a great deal of self-confidence. It had had 10 years of increasing prosperity, a flourishing base of heavy industry and a stable society in which all "knew their place".

But there were already clouds on the horizon. The Boer War, at the beginning of the century, had shown that the military might, so successful in dealing with ill-equipped groups in Africa and India, was rather less effective in coping with a well-armed, determined, although much smaller and poorer, group of white settlers. The ruling classes had also been shocked by the rejection of 34% of volunteers because of their poor physical condition. But change had begun. The 1906 Education Act empowered local authorities to provide school meals for needy children and the 1911 National Insurance Act provided a system of insurance against ill health for a large section of the working population, within certain age and financial limits.

The immense sacrifices of the country during World War I had serious consequences for society. Much of the country's wealth had been spent on the war effort and Britain was much poorer afterwards. The returning soldiers expected to find a better society, with full employment, and were gravely disappointed by the reality. Many heavy industries, such as coal, steel, shipbuilding and railways, had been exploited to the full during wartime. As a result, by the end, they were often run-down and much less productive than similar industries built up in the United States to cope with the war.

Appendix 1 lists the various governments by political party, the Prime Ministers and the percentage of unemployed. This 20-year period saw the eclipse of the Liberal Party and the rise of Labour. The latter held office for short periods, on their own on two occasions and with Conservatives in the National Governments after 1931. This led to a split within the Labour party which was only healed after World War II. The political background to this period is well described in books such as those by Marwick,[1] Taylor,[2] Laybourn,[3] and Jenkins.[4]

Unemployment and the Depression were dominant themes which influenced all activities throughout this period. There was an inexorable rise in unemployment to 1931, with only a relatively small diminution up to the beginning of World War II. The distribution of unemployment was uneven both between trades – for example, 60% of shipbuilders, 41% of coal miners, 31% of cotton workers – and between regions – for example, 13.7% in London and the Southeast, 27% in the North, Northeast and Northwest, and 36.5% in Wales. All governments tried to extend the provisions of benefit to the unemployed but the amount of benefit had to be reduced at the time of the Depression and this resulted in much hardship for many.

Although all governments accepted that the cash benefits for the unemployed were inadequate, they excused this on grounds of economic difficulties. Newman, the Chief Medical Officer of the day, undertook a series of surveys of the health of the population in areas of high unemployment and concluded that there was little evidence of harm. As Lewis Fanning,[5] a young epidemiologist, showed, it was unlikely that conditions for people living in areas of long-term deprivation could get much worse. The findings of these official studies, however, were very different from the conclusions drawn by independent workers such as Orr[6] and M'Gonigle.[7]

The effects of World War I had also contributed to the Russian Revolution and the advent of communism. This influenced attitudes in the United Kingdom. Firstly, there was a great fear, especially among the better-off, that a similar situation might arise in the UK. This is well illustrated by the results of the November 1924 elections in which the spectre of the "Red menace" was raised by publication of a forged letter purporting to come from Zinoviev, Secretary of the Russian Communist Party. Organised trade unions were also afraid of being taken over by the Communists. Secondly, the working classes were dissatisfied with the high rate of unemployment and the conditions of work prevailing after the war. This led to numerous strikes and culminated in the General Strike of 1926.

Many authors, of whom Orwell[8] is probably the best known, have commented that England was two, three or four nations. JB Priestley[9] focused on the differences between the England of "Cathedrals and Minsters" and industrial England. He suggested that the distinctions were more than those between occupational groups and contended that there were differing impacts in different places of the variations in income, status and economic prosperity. These descriptions epitomised the class divisions and tensions which existed in society at the time, in a climate that was very different from the expectations of the soldiers who had endured great hardship during the war and expected a better life at its end.

One of the main preoccupations of government was housing. "Housing for Heroes" had been a universal promise immediately after the end of the war. Christopher Addison, Minister of Health and also responsible for housing in 1918, was energetic in promoting the building of new houses and renting them at controlled rents. Lloyd George, however, considered Addison profligate in his policies, and forced him to resign in 1921. Addison's successors – Sir Arthur Mond, Griffith Boscowen and Neville Chamberlain – continued the policy of building new homes but standards and quality were sharply reduced to make them more affordable within available public resources.

As already mentioned, the major preoccupation at this time of high unemployment was with the Depression and the fear of communism. Although there was some concern with the problems of poverty – particularly by charitable bodies including the Joseph Rowntree Foundation – there was little concerted effort to deal with these.

Political allegiances in the UK between the wars was split between, on the one hand, the ideas of the right wing and, on the other, Keynesian (Liberal) concepts and the left as represented by Keir Hardie and the Independent Labour Party and later by Foot and Bevin who were also at odds with the Communists. By contrast in the United States – where there was also a difference of focus between the Conservative (Republican) and Liberal (Democrat) parties – the response to such events as the Depression was far more radical.

This difference had an effect on the type of EPHR being carried out. Before World War I, EPHR in both countries was largely concerned with the prevention of infectious disease and the study of vital statistics.[10] After the war, however, EPHR and medical research in general received greater academic support in the US than in the UK.[11] Approaches to the solution of public health problems were also more radical in the US. They tackled the underlying causes of these problems rather than concentrating on mechanisms and superficial symptoms. At this time, of course, a large part of the map of the world was coloured red – for the British Empire – and this undoubtedly reinforced attitudes of self-satisfaction and self-reliance on this side of the Atlantic. This lack of concern with what was happening outside the British Isles was demonstrated by the widespread neglect of events in the rest of Europe – the growth of Nazism and the political and social chaos in France – until it was almost too late. This undoubtedly had an effect on the environment in which EPHR was practised and the questions which it tackled in the UK.

But, although politics and society in the US seemed more aware of and concerned with the effects of the Depression and unemployment, the US was also profoundly isolationist in its attitudes and policies in relation to the rest of the world at this time. However, although society in both countries still considered social Darwinism or survival of the fittest as a solution, individual charitable giving and action was more marked in the US. Charitable foundations were certainly more active there in the support of academic institutions. A good example of this was the support given to academic medicine and public health by the Rockefeller Foundation at Johns Hopkins University.[11]

The Rockefeller Foundation, however, did not limit its concern with public health to the US, but was also responsible for the foundation of Schools or Departments of Public Health in London, Rio de Janeiro and Peking.[12]

No British charity or individual supported EPHR similarly. Foundations such as Rowntree and Cadbury were concerned with the alleviation of poverty but did not consider EPHR as a suitable vehicle for their concerns. The question of the differences in charitable support between the two countries is not central to this work but is worth noting in any analysis of EPHR.

The era between the two World Wars was profoundly schismatic. On the one hand there were those that prospered and lived as an enclosed group, ignoring what was going on around them. The results of poverty hardly impinged on their lives and consciousness. Their desire was to return to the certainties that existed before 1914 and to believe in the invincibility of "the Empire". At the same time they feared the growth of communism, radical ideas and many of the changes in attitudes and behaviour. They believed in the capability of the able to prosper, and were concerned with alleviating the effects of poverty. This group felt that they should be rewarded and not punished for all the deaths, damages and deprivations of the war.

On the other hand, there were those who were profoundly affected by the Depression, were unemployed, had suffered as much, or more, in the war and considered that unless there was a definite move from the pre-war status quo, no change for the better would be possible. Many in this group were now educated, and as a result of war service had seen life outside their village or town and had mixed with individuals from differing backgrounds for the first time in their lives.

This divide in British society was reflected in the attitudes to and conduct of EPHR. Medical schools were almost entirely run by hospital consultants; medical research of all forms, and not only EPHR, was a poor relation of medical practice. Only a few courageous individuals, such as M'Gonigle and Boyd Orr, actually tried to challenge this state of affairs. Those in control of research – for example, the Medical Research Council – were loath to challenge those in authority by supporting research which might make uncomfortable reading, or help in the understanding of the mechanisms of disease but not in correcting the fundamental causes. In these conditions it is not particularly surprising that EPHR in this period did not flourish.

THE UNITED STATES 1919–1939

The end of World War I found America in a completely different situation from that prevailing in the United Kingdom.

America had entered the twentieth century with a great deal of optimism and many of the wounds of the Civil War had healed. The Industrial Revolution, which started in the second decade of the nineteenth century, began to have an effect by 1880 when the value of manufactured products surpassed that of agricultural products and more people derived their livelihood from industry rather than farming. This industrialisation was accompanied by increasing prosperity, urbanisation and improvement in access to education. On the downside was the emergence of huge corporations with their power to control labour and prices, continuing colour discrimination, and an increase in the gap between rich and poor. The beginning of the twentieth century also saw America accepting world power status and shedding the anti-military, anti-imperial tradition. This was probably largely the result of a need for foreign markets but also of the American military victories in the 113-day Spanish-American War in 1898. But, for all the public contentment, at the turn of the century, many so-called progressives were seeking reform.

The progressives were united in their desire to right the wrongs caused by industrialisation, urbanisation and immigration, although they agreed about the inherent value of capitalism, private property, democracy and individual freedom. Most reformers believed that the power of government could accomplish their ends. These beliefs dominated American life for the rest of the century and influenced the New Deal, the Fair Deal, the New Frontier, the Great Society and other such movements.

In the late nineteenth century many state legislatures were dominated by political "bosses". Reformers recognised that their effectiveness would be reduced unless there was an improvement in the quality of state politics. The first success in this endeavour was the election of Robert M La Follette as governor of Wisconsin in 1900.

When President William McKinley was assassinated in 1901 he was succeeded by Theodore Roosevelt who became the leading proponent of the reformers. He recognised the need for America to play a role in international affairs. In spite of his own great wealth most of his sympathies and actions were directed to curbing the power of rich industrialists and to helping the trade unions.

Roosevelt was succeeded by William Taft in 1909. He was not considered an effective President, partly because of his conservatism in an age of reform, and he in turn was succeeded in 1913 by Woodrow Wilson, a Democrat.

By 1914 Wilson had retreated from his progressive policies. This was perhaps partly because of a minor recession and the opposition of the Republicans to his tariff and anti-trust policies. But although progress for reform was less in later years, the seeds had been sown.

Almost all Americans wanted to keep America out of World War I, and Wilson declared neutrality in 1914, but opinions soon began to change. Public sympathies and economic and industrial ties were with the Allies. All segments of the economy began to prosper. Wilson was re-elected President and in 1917 declared war on Germany after a series of provocations caused by U-boats sinking American vessels bound for Europe.

The war forced the American government to exercise unprecedented power over the economy and to raise taxes. But the war also had a major beneficial effect in stimulating growth in the output of all industries as well as agriculture. Workers benefited and many groups such as women and black people found employment and were crucial to the war effort. American losses were far less than those of its European Allies – there were, for example, about 112 000 dead (more than half from disease) compared to about one million British casualties.

The war did not have the profound social effects on America that were seen in the UK but there were some similarities. Immediately after the end of the war, for example, labour disturbances increased for a time, and although there were only about 70 000 Communists (less than 0.1% of the population) there was a transient "Red scare".

Between 1922 and 1929 industrial output nearly doubled and although not everyone shared in the increase in prosperity, millions of Americans were able to enjoy a standard of living that was barely imaginable before 1914. Mass production dominated the economy, exemplified by the motor car. Prosperity enabled millions of young people to stay at school and all 48 states had compulsory education laws, many effective up to the age of 18 years. The introduction of laws to prohibit the sale of alcohol (until 1933) was one manifestation of the fundamentalism in many parts of society.

The 1920s were dominated by the Republican Party. Harding won the 1920 election, died in office in 1923, and was succeeded by Coolidge, who was succeeded by Herbert Hoover in 1928. This era was relatively calm. The US enjoyed peace and unprecedented prosperity. It was interspersed by a number of scandals of corruption and a return to isolationist attitudes. The administrations helped corporations at the expense of labour unions.

Hoover presided over the start of the Depression. There are many explanations for the cataclysmic events on the New York Stock Exchange in October 1929 which triggered the Great Depression of the 1930s. Undoubtedly the unequal distribution of income limited the number of customers for the products of mass production, corporate structure deficits enabled the unscrupulous to speculate with other people's money and erect pyramids of no value, and finally an unfavourable balance of trade probably also contributed to the collapse. The economy both urban and rural declined disastrously.

By 1932 about 25% of the population was unemployed, with rates of 50% in Cleveland and 80% in Toledo. Unemployment compensation was only introduced in 1932, in Wisconsin. Hoover tried to help, by exuding optimism, encouraging easy credit and expanding a federal work programme. There were one or two episodes of industrial unrest – 20 000 unemployed veterans, for example, marched on Washington in June–July 1932, but in general, most of the country continued to trust the nation's political and economic institutions.

Roosevelt won the 1932 election with a sweeping victory. He and his advisers approached their task in a way which reflected the reform tradition. Their concern for the poor rested on the "Social Gospel" and they were confident about the power of federal government. Many had worked with the poor in settlement houses in the cities. Their policies were directed to alleviating problems of deprivation and encouraging the revival of the economy.

One example of this was the initial temporary closure of all banks, followed by reform and guarantee of deposits in those considered viable. Farmers were paid to take land out of production and thus reduce the problems of over-production. Fair competition rules were introduced in business and in its dealings with labour. A public works administration put people to work – building libraries, parks, hospitals and bridges. Since many families had lost their homes, measures were taken to provide the necessary finance to help in obtaining housing.

Roosevelt was re-elected in 1936 for a second term, with an even greater majority. The impetus for the New Deal, as it was called, gradually diminished. It had been opposed by many wealthy conservative Republicans. But the reformers were not helped by labour violence, particularly in 1937, involving one of the main unions. The New Deal did not end the Great Depression.

A decade after the Stock Market crash there were still about 10 million unemployed out of a labour pool of 40 million. Nonetheless it had helped many, enabled business and the economy to recover, encouraged the rise of organised labour, introduced unemployment insurance and old age pensions and improved housing tenure, electricity supply and education. It was not until World War II started that a full recovery was seen.

Throughout this period private agencies and funds played a very active role, not only in the alleviation of the effects of poverty and inequalities of income but also in the support of institutions involved in research and the provision of services, including education, intended to correct or modify the effects of poverty. "From 1900 to 1940 the influence of private agencies and funds was stronger than that of the federal government in health research, owing largely to the impact of those extraordinary organisations established by John D Rockefeller during the first two decades of the century – the Rockefeller Institute, the Rockefeller Foundation, and the General Education Board."[13] Many wealthy individuals, such as Carnegie, Duke, Milbank and Josiah Macy, followed in Rockefeller's footsteps. This philanthropy was largely possible because of the vast surplus of wealth which had accumulated by 1930.

THE UNITED KINGDOM 1945–1979
In spite of the enormous casualties and economic and social effects of World War I, little effort had been made during its course to plan what would happen when it ended. The sacrifices of the population were expected and acknowledged. For those in power, life before 1914 had been good and they expected that conditions after the war ended would revert to those prevailing before.

Events between the two wars challenged this attitude, and although the rise of socialism, the trade unions and communism in Russia had been contained, the threats of fascism in Germany and Italy and their acquisitive policies were accepted by many as an even greater threat.

Britain entered the war with very recent memories of poverty and unemployment. In 1940, after the fall of France, there was a real prospect of defeat which did not diminish until 1943–44. The Government had learned from the mistakes of 1914–1918. The U-boats and the need to produce munitions in World War I had reduced the availability of food. England before

1945 depended on its Empire for many essential foodstuffs and was unable to satisfy demand through local production. This led, in World War I, to a hurriedly devised inefficient method of food rationing. In 1939–40, by contrast, rationing was introduced as a planned measure and sufficient and adequate amounts were distributed equitably at a price that all could afford. Omitting bread from being rationed ensured that no one went hungry. The principles of this scheme were based on the findings of Boyd Orr[6] and have been described elsewhere.[10]

Most important of all, however, was the recognition that it was necessary to give the population hope that if the war was won, life would be better than it had been previously.

As a result, the wartime Government embarked on planning a variety of improvements in social policy, education, housing and above all employment which would be introduced if the war was won. The Beveridge Report (1942) was a prime example of this.

Labour won the election in 1945 with an overwhelming majority. Although the parties in power changed several times between 1945 and 1979 the majorities achieved were never so large again. This period has been labelled as the "Consensus Period",[1] and there were certain constant themes throughout:

- There was a belief that government intervention was beneficial and necessary in order to increase national stability, improve economic performance, and ensure growth in the economy.

- The desire for economic stability and growth was paramount. This was considered achievable through the use of fiscal policies such as taxation, subsidies and control of development.

- There needed to be a public social policy to cope with the effects of unemployment, the elderly (pensions), children, the disabled, and later even termination of pregnancy.

- The distinctions between the social classes were reduced, particularly by improving both access to and quality of education at all levels of society from primary to higher education.

- The epitome of these general social themes was the introduction of the National Health Service which was to provide comprehensive health and rehabilitation services for the prevention and cure of disease and restoration of capacity for work, available to all members of the community.

- The decline of the Empire and Britain's role in the colonies was accepted, with a concomitant rise in concern with European affairs.

Labour's electoral victory in 1945 ensured that priority was given to the social aspects of the above-mentioned themes. The National Health Service was introduced in 1948. It is, however, important to note that most of the public health services were not included in the changes until 1974.[10] Of greatest importance, however, was the maintenance of full employment, a feature of war. Basic industries – coal, steel and transport – were nationalised. Rationing of food, clothes and furniture persisted for some years – food until the 1950s. Economic problems soon appeared, partly because of the inability of our industries to compete with others overseas that had not been destroyed or affected by the war and also because other countries developed industries that competed with our own. The wartime destruction of some of the docks and the lack of adequate maintenance of those that survived meant that the UK was unable to import or export efficiently.

The main problem was that the UK was living beyond its means, and yet considered itself still as a major imperial power. The wealth built up before 1939 had been spent waging war, and loans and help from the US were no longer forthcoming. The Korean War, some colonial conflicts such as those in Malaya, Kenya and Palestine, and the maintenance of some large overseas bases – for example, in Aden and Singapore – contributed to the economic problems of this period.

The fall of Germany and rise of the two superpowers, Russia and the United States, had a profound impact on the beliefs and concepts of UK governments. It became accepted that the UK alone could not have a major international role but could have an influence internationally in combination with others.

The loss of imperial influence and concern meant that greater attention began to be paid to domestic matters such as health, education, employment, environment and other social and economic policies. Economic growth rates were high and unemployment was low.

Increasing prosperity permeated to all groups. There was a substantial increase in house ownership, cars, telephones and televisions. This was a period of great technological innovation in medicine and in other fields of life with, for example, the introduction of detergents and frozen foods. The population was optimistic and expected (and largely attained) a better life and conditions year on year. The Welfare State ensured that people felt secure, even if they became ill or unemployed. Social benefits, such as children's allowances, ensured that even the most deprived had an income sufficient for basic needs. Direct taxes (income tax) were relatively high, particularly for the rich; indirect taxes, such as purchase tax (now VAT) relatively low. Disparity in income between social class groups began to diminish gradually.

Although industrial strife was common, particularly among coal miners and railway workers, relations between social groups was improving. Education, particularly in universities, expanded. Three new medical schools were founded, at Southampton, Leicester and Nottingham. Medical research grew, as did public health and epidemiological departments, then called Social Medicine. Research in these subjects became less uncommon although this growth was uneven. New areas of concern, such as the molecular sciences and health services research, began to emerge.

With increasing prosperity, more resources became available for health, social services and education. The increase in resources for the NHS was epitomised by the beginning of a planned programme of rebuilding of hospitals. At this time the split between clinical services provided in hospitals, general medical services provided by GPs, and preventive and public health services provided by local authorities began to be questioned. After an eight-year period of gestation and consultation all three services were united under one Area Health Authority in 1974.[10] For EPHR it was hoped that union would improve the quantity and quality of relevant research, and the ability to undertake it.

The 1973 oil price rise, associated with the Arab–Israeli War, represented the end of this period of growth of government intervention, economic stability, and growth of social policies including concerns with the health service and medical research and education. Although there is no doubt that there has been an increasing concern with social policies such as education, health, and welfare benefits since that time, until 2000 there has not been a continuing commitment to improvement in the services provided on a national basis. Most of the author's contemporaries look back on the 60s and early 70s with nostalgia as things always improved year on year.

Part of the reason for this change in atmosphere was the decline in the economy and major problems with balance of payments. There was an increase in industrial disputes and strikes, particularly among public sector workers. But also, consensus politics was no longer acceptable. The Conservative Party, under Margaret Thatcher shifted to the right with market-oriented policies, abandoning the politics of consensus, while the Labour Party disintegrated into two groups: left-wing and centre. It was thus not surprising that Labour lost the election in 1979, and that Margaret Thatcher gained power with a large parliamentary majority.

THE UNITED STATES 1945–1979

When World War II ended, America was once again in a different position from that of the UK, as it had been after World War I. There was no physical damage and the economy was strong – far stronger than in 1939. The returning soldiers wished to enjoy the products available, such as cars, televisions and washing machines. Roosevelt had died in office in 1945 and was succeeded by Truman. He had to cope with a conservative Congress, soaring inflation and militant trade unions. Anti-communism dominated Washington politics. There were few additions to the social programmes initiated before the war. Truman won the election of 1948 but his term of office was dominated by the Korean War and increasing fear of "Reds" (McCarthyism). Since Congress was dominated by conservatives, little was achieved in the way of social legislation, although there was a rise in the minimum wage and in social security benefits.

The major issues dominating the presidency of Eisenhower (1953–1961) were:

- The ending of the "Red Scare" and disenchantment with McCarthy and his followers.

- Increasing prosperity and growth of the economy with no redistribution of wealth. By 1960 it is estimated that between one-fifth and one-quarter of the population could not survive on their earned income.[14] Unemployment, however, was 3% or less.

- In 1954 a ground-breaking civil rights decision was reached which ruled that segregated public schools were illegal.

- Since the US had few foreign possessions, colonial problems did not exist. But the imperatives of the Cold War and containment of Russian interests meant that the US became involved in a wide variety of imperial conflicts in the Middle East and Asia, and was involved in the development of a major military arsenal.

Kennedy succeeded Eisenhower in 1961. He was assassinated in 1963 and was in turn succeeded by his Vice President, Johnson, who remained in power until 1969. This period, which started with high hopes for a variety of social reforms, did not achieve its objectives – largely because of the US's involvement in the Vietnam War. The main themes during this era were:

- Continuing obsession with anti-communism which led to a number of foreign policy interventions, such as the Cuban missile crisis, Bay of Pigs, Berlin, and involvement in South-East Asia–Vietnam in particular.

- Introduction of Medicare, which provides health care for most people aged 65 years and over.

- Introduction of Medicaid to provide medical and dental care for low-income Americans.

- The provision of federal aid to help students in public and parochial schools.

- The introduction of a series of Civil Rights Acts which, among other measures, outlawed poll taxes.

What is most remembered about this era, however, is US involvement in a war in Vietnam. This was the cause of great division in the American people, with large-scale anti-war demonstrations. In general, it was the young who opposed US involvement in Vietnam. Many of them associated the war with capitalism and racial intolerance. During this period the churches also began to develop greater influence and the growth of feminism was marked.

Nixon won the election in 1969. He was forced to resign in 1973 because of the Watergate scandal and was succeeded by Ford. The major issues at this time were the effort to disengage from the conflict in Vietnam, the attempt to establish relations with China, and the beginnings of a dialogue with Russia. Little was achieved in reforms of welfare although racial integration policies continued to be pursued.

THE UNITED KINGDOM 1979–1999

The first 25 years after World War II were marked in Britain by a spirit of optimism, growth in the economy and a concern for social welfare. This was exemplified by the introduction of and support for the National Health Service and expansion of education generally and universities in particular. This had a marked effect on both the quality and the quantity of epidemiological public health research which was, at last, becoming a respectable and important field. The last few years of this period, however, were beginning to be marked by doubt, a disappearance of the spirit of optimism, and economic problems. Unemployment increased, university and research funding began to be cut back (or at least did not grow at the same pace) and questioning of the principles and policies of the Welfare State began to receive publicity.

The advent of the Conservative administration in 1979 marked the beginning of 18 continuous years of Conservative rule. These years were accompanied by major events in other parts of the world – the Falklands War, the Gulf War, strife in the Balkans and Africa, but above all the collapse of communism in 1989.

The main themes of the 18 years of Conservative rule represented marked changes in rhetoric, as well as in policies.

There was gradual dismantling of almost all the nationalised industries – for example, coal, steel, railways, telephones and electricity generation and distribution – by sale to the private sector. This contributed to an increase in the participation of many in buying and selling shares on the Stock Market.

Major curbs to the power of the trade unions and the possible disruption of services were put in place.

Attacks on what were considered to be examples of the Welfare State were made, including the sale of council homes which has contributed to homeless people on the streets, virtually unknown since the 1930s.

Some welfare benefits began to be reduced and there was political rhetoric to reduce the central power of the state. State expenditure in fact changed little. Centralised authority was enhanced by the reduction in the power of elected local authorities, and in the NHS there was an increase in central direction and a corresponding diminution in local decision-making.[15]

Direct taxes were reduced radically, particularly for the more affluent, while indirect taxation increased. This led to a resurgence of the growth in the gap between the rich and the poor. It should, however, be noted that the total proportion of tax collected remained virtually static.

Manufacturing industry declined very markedly so that by the end of the twentieth century, few heavy industries, such as coal, steel, and shipbuilding, survived. This was accompanied by a great deal of unemployment, particularly in the former industrial areas such as Wales, the Northeast and Northwest of England, and throughout Scotland. At the same time there has been considerable growth in service industries, such as information technology and financial services. This has been particularly concentrated in the Southeast, increasing the North–South divide, in terms of both income and employment.

During this period there was a great deal of industrial unrest, particularly among coal miners and groups of unskilled workers such as postmen. The change in emphasis of where and how people were employed and the increase in the need for unskilled manual labour accompanied by the privatisation of services (contracting out) in local authorities and the NHS changed both the quality and the commitment of workers in these enterprises for the worse.

There had been a great deal of immigration to the UK, beginning in the 40s and 50s from the Caribbean and in the 70s and 80s from the Far East, India, Pakistan and Bangladesh. This led to many parts of the UK becoming multiracial communities where immigrants usually settled in the degenerating areas of inner cities, often in grossly inadequate premises. They were likely to be unemployed or in intermittent, badly paid work as, for example, cleaners in hospitals.

A major change in the attitudes of the population, now encouraged by government, was the growth in consumerism with increased expectations of what public services, particularly those by bodies such as the NHS, could and should deliver. This was promoted by the introduction of consumer charters or guarantees of a level of service to be accepted. Unfortunately, these charters were rarely accompanied by the extra resources required to meet them; instead it was expected that "efficiency gains" should be made. The emphasis on individual rights, often at the expense of the public good, has led to a marked increase in compensation litigation for medical errors, medical negligence, administrative mistakes, employment practice and the like.

Changes in educational policy affected both schools and higher education. In the former, the educational principles of the 1960s, based on the idea that children should discover for themselves, began to be questioned, with reintroduction of rigid schedules in the basic aspects of reading, writing and mathematics and the introduction of national examinations at set ages as well as regular national school inspections. In higher education, most of the institutes and technical colleges which had been under local authority control were redefined as universities and became the responsibility of a higher education funding council under central control. Bureaucratic methods of assessment of teaching quality and research quality and productivity were introduced. Resources for research, including EPHR, were reduced, as were the resources for higher education.

The attitudes of Government to EPHR were ambiguous. Research funding shared the cuts imposed on all educational and welfare services. When a highly emotive epidemic of AIDS arose, however, there was no shortage of funding for research, particularly that concerned with treatment and the development of a vaccine. The fundamental behavioural survey required to assess possible preventive measures by assessing sexual attitudes and behaviours was not funded by Government but by a private charity.[16] Other relevant research on social problems was not encouraged. Perhaps the best example of this was seen in the area of inequalities in health. This had first been tackled by the Black Report.[17] No notice was taken of its findings, the minister stated that "the solutions proposed are too costly and not proven", and no follow-up research was commissioned. In 1994 the Government commissioned a further report[18] which found that such inequalities were due to a variety of causes including environment, social and genetic factors. Poverty was not referred to. It is shaming that some of the social scientists and epidemiologists involved in preparing this report did not have the courage to speak plainly against the Government position. When the Blair administration came to power one of their first tasks was to tackle this problem.[19] The Acheson Report, with some of the same cast as the previous report, blamed mainly poverty and the increasing disparity in income and facilities between social classes and different areas over the past 18 years for increasing health inequalities.

Major changes to the NHS in management, structure and organisation were introduced in the period 1989–1991.[15] These involved the separation of providers of services (hospitals) from the purchasers of services (authorities and general practitioners). Alterations in the method of funding general practice were also introduced. These changes were introduced on the basis of the beliefs of Ministers and their advisers and civil servants without reference to previous research findings or acknowledgement of the need to evaluate whether the changes actually delivered what was promised. This, in many respects, epitomised the change in attitude towards social or population research: it was not essential and could easily be replaced by authoritarian opinion based on experiences in a completely different field. The neglect of epidemiological public health research in particular and research in general at this time was the subject of a House of Lords inquiry.[20]

Perhaps the most important event in this time period, however, was the collapse of Communism. This resulted in the radical left (Bennite) faction of the Labour party losing most of its influence and made the Left (New Labour) once more electable. As shown in the table, Labour was re-elected in 1997. As a result, investment in social policy again became possible.

Nonetheless, two aspects of the old society persist. Class differences remain and inequalities in the distribution of wealth are greater than at any time since 1929. The rise in consumerism, personal expectations and emphasis on individual solutions are a permanent heritage of the Thatcher years.

The UK has lost its Empire and has become a multiracial society. It is difficult, at this time, to make any judgment on the influence of EPHR under the Labour Government. The Labour administration's concern with health inequalities and poverty have been associated with some increase in research in this field. More money has been put into health and education services, and researchers are no longer threatened by year-on-year reduction in resources. But it is still noticeable that the ground gained by EPHR in the period 1945–1979 and lost in the last 20 years, has not been regained. Unfortunately, the lack of concern by the NHS for health services research noted by the House of Lords in 1988[20] is still evident at the beginning of the twenty-first century.

THE UNITED STATES 1979–1999

The end of the Carter presidency was marked by some disillusionment with government and its politics. This has been described as "a crisis of confidence in government".[21] Carter's image had been gravely compromised by his handling of the Iran hostage crisis and the economy. This was an unfortunate ending to what had started with some optimism. Carter had begun with the ambition to restore integrity to the White House, to balance the budget and to end waste in government. The American electorate did not have great faith in his leadership – this was confirmed in his years in office when he demonstrated his integrity and diligence but a lack of vision.

A revolution in Iran against the unpopular, corrupt pro-American regime of the Shah had resulted in the access to power of an intransigent, orthodox clerical administration with very marked anti-Western, anti-American policies. As a result of these, Iran – the second largest exporter of oil – stopped the flow of oil from its wells to the West, causing a huge increase in world oil prices. The anti-American slant of the regime was also demonstrated in an attack on the US Embassy during which some of its staff were held hostage. Carter's administration was considered inept in the handling of these events.

When Carter took office America was just beginning to recover from a period of recession which had started in the Ford years. In 1977 the unemployment rate was about 8 per cent and the rate of inflation about 6 per cent. By 1980 the former had fallen to 6 per cent but the latter had risen to 13 per cent.[14] The reduction in oil supply from Iran led to major increases in the cost of heating oil and petroleum which exacerbated the economic problems.

Reagan won the election of 1980 with a substantial majority. At the start of his period in office the economy was flagging, and there was marked inflation and a huge budget deficit. Reagan had very conservative principles – and did his best to implement these, largely through the work of his appointees. He himself enjoyed his years in power, but "paid little attention to the work of government, took frequent vacations, and was known by insiders to be intellectually as well as physically lazy".[14]

He was re-elected convincingly for a second term of office by a huge majority. He had little interest in social issues, and in spite of increasing disparities between the rich and the poor did not hesitate to promote cuts to food stamps and school lunch programmes. He was very concerned to reduce federal expenditures. At the same time his conservative policies led to lower taxes, particularly for the more affluent.

Prosperity began to return to America in 1983–84, gross national product grew, new jobs were created and inflation fell. There was marked enthusiasm for Reagan's economic policies. This period was also marked by a number of other events. From the public health viewpoint the most important of these were the appearance of the AIDS epidemic and the development of computing technology to create what became known as the information superhighway. Both these factors helped to increase interest in and expenditure on health research.

Perhaps of greater future significance was a realisation of the decline of standards of education, particularly in schools, which was considered to be a local or state problem and not a federal concern. At the same time there was a rise in the crime rate, particularly of violent crimes. The prison population was increased, many being imprisoned for drug-related crimes.

One of the most important events during Reagan's Presidency was the rapprochement with the Soviet Union. At the start of his period in office, relations were fraught; towards the end he had come to an accommodation with Gorbachev. Two other foreign adventures had less happy outcomes. The first was the bombing of Libya on suspicion of its involvement in terrorist acts; the second was a series of scandals related to unauthorised support of reactionary governments in Central America, particularly Nicaragua.

Reagan left office in 1989 with an unprecedented approval rating. The economy was thriving and communism was "on the run". The Cold War was over. It was thus not surprising that Reagan's Vice President, George Bush, was elected to the Presidency. Bush was very different from Reagan although he continued to develop many conservative policies. The major events at this time were the Persian Gulf War. Iraq invaded Kuwait in August 1990; America and its allies opposed this and defeated Iraq in February 1991. Problems with China, and its human rights policies, replaced concern with the Soviet Union. Domestically, episodes of racial conflict marked Bush's term of office.

Bush was succeeded by a Democrat, Bill Clinton in 1993. Over the next eight years this administration presided over a growing economy and increasing prosperity. A major initiative on universal health insurance met with great opposition and failed to be introduced. There were a number of sexual scandals implicating the President, while his wife was accused of financial conflicts of interest. Foreign affairs were dominated by the problems of the break-up of Yugoslavia and increasing tension in the Middle East.

As Roberts[23] has stated, at the end of the decade the US was "more of the same". Even after a cavalier piling up of debt the economy was strong and prosperous. There was great dynamism in the country, in spite of all the social and political conservatism, as shown by 7 million people changing state and one-fifth moving house annually.[22] Black people were better off than ever before – but in spite of increasing prosperity, more individuals were economically deprived and this was coming to be recognised. Clinton was not blamed for the lack of progress on the domestic front but for the dissipation of presidential authority due to the sexual scandals during his Presidency.

Conclusion

Description of the salient events and trends in the politics of the UK and USA and in the concerns of our two societies has highlighted some major common trends and issues. In both countries the problems of poverty and deprivation have dominated the scene at different times. Between the two World Wars unemployment and poverty was an issue in both countries. It was striking that in the UK this affected social, geographic and occupational groups in a selective manner, whereas the Depression in the USA was a far more general phenomenon from which few areas or groups were exempt. After World War II the problems of unemployment and poverty persisted, but in both countries it was usually localised to specific areas or ethnic groups. A general phenomenon has been the increasing inequalities between different groups, with simultaneous improvement in both health and economic status of all groups.

In both countries the demise of communism has been one of the major changes in the political landscape. It has not been our task to analyse the major political and historical forces in the twentieth century but to examine whether there have been changes in our societies that have affected the commissioning of EPHR.

Before 1939 specific state funding for health research was sparse. In the United States, private charitable foundations were very generous in supporting the relevant institutions and research in both countries. Most other research was founded by the MRC in the UK and through the USPHS in the USA.

After World War II, funding in both the US and UK became much more readily available from federal sources such as NIH in the US and from state sources such as the MRC and Department of Health in the UK. There has, however, been a change in attitude towards research (and life generally) in the USA which, as Sandel[23] describes, has replaced old attitudes. This is beginning to occur in the UK as well. This attitude "asserts the priority of the rights over the good".[23] The American concept of welfare is thus not based on the European ethic of civic or communal obligation (solidarity) but on the concept of freedom – that is, the right of each individual to choose his or her own values and ends.

These attitudes help us to understand some of the differences which are seen in the direction and content of EPHR in the two countries and, most importantly, indicate the obstacles faced by epidemiologists and public health researchers in both countries whose major motivation is to improve the lot of the population as a whole – and of the deprived above all.

REFERENCES

1 Marwick A. (2000) *A History of the Modern British Isles 1914 1999.* Oxford: Blackwell.

2 Taylor AJP. (1992) *English History 1914–1945.* Oxford: Oxford University Press.

3 Laybourn K. (1990) *Britain on the Breadline 1918–1939.* Stroud: Sutton Publishing.

4 Jenkins R. (1995) *Baldwin.* London: Macmillan.

5 Lewis Fanning E. (1937) A study of the trend of mortality rates in urban communities of England and Wales with specific reference to depressed areas. *Lancet*, 1: 865–867.

6 Orr JB. (1936) *Food, Health and Income.* London: Macmillan.

7 M'Gonigle GCM, Kirby J. (1936) *Poverty and Public Health.* London: Victor Gollancz.

8 Orwell G. (1937) *The Road to Wigan Pier.* London: Victor Gollancz.

9 Priestley JB. (1934) *English Journey.* London: Heinemann.

10 Holland WW, Stewart S. (1998) *Public Health – The Vision and the Challenge.* London: Nuffield Trust.

11 Fee E. (1987) *Disease and Discovery.* Baltimore, MD: Johns Hopkins University Press.

12 Fee E, Acheson RM. (1991) *A History of Education in Public Health.* London: Oxford Medical Publishing.

13 Rosen G. (1965) Patterns of Health Research in the United States 1900–1960. *Bulletin of the History of Medicine*, 39: 201–221.

14 Reeves TC. (2000) *Twentieth Century America*. Oxford: Oxford University Press.

15 Kember T, Macpherson G. (1994) *The NHS – a Kaleidoscope of Care – Conflicts of Service and Business Values*. London: Nuffield Provincial Hospitals Trust.

16 Johnson AM, Wadsworth J, Wellings K, Field J. (1994) *Sexual Attitudes and Lifestyles*. Oxford: Blackwell Scientific.

17 *Inequalities in health* (The Black Report) 1980. London: DHSS.

18 DHSS. (1998) *Variations in Health. What Can the Department of Health and the NHS Do?* London: HMSO.

19 DHSS. (1998) *Independent Inquiry into Inequalities in Health* (Acheson Report). London: HMSO.

20 House of Lords Select Committee on Science and Technology. (1988) *Priorities in Medical Research*. Vol. 1. Report HL 54-I. London: HMSO.

21 Diggins JP. (1997) *The Liberal Persuasion: Arthur Schlesiger Jnr, and the Challenge of the American Past*. Princeton, NJ: Princeton University Press.

22 Roberts JM. (1999) *The Penguin History of the Twentieth Century*. London: Penguin Books.

23 Sandel MJ. (1996) *Democracy's Discontent: America in Search of a Public Philosophy*. Cambridge, MA: Belknap Press of Harvard University Press.

APPENDIX 1

Gen. Election	Party	Prime Minister	Voting			Unemployment
Date			*Party*	*Number*	*Seats*	
1918 December	Coalition	Lloyd George	Coalition	5 121 000	478	Not known
			Conservative	663 000	48	
			Labour	2 385 000	63	
			Liberal	1 299 000	28	
			Sinn Fein	487 000	73	
1922 November	Conservative	Bonar Law	Conservative	5 400 000	345	
		Stanley Baldwin	Liberal	4 000 000	117	1 540 000 (15.2%)
			Labour	4 200 000	142	1 275 000 (11.3%)
1924 January	Labour	Ramsey MacDonald	Conservative	5 400 000	258	1 130 000 (10.9%)
			Liberal	4 200 000	159	
			Labour	4 300 000	40	
1924 November	Conservative	Stanley Baldwin	Conservative	8 000 000	419	1 226 000 (11.2%)
			Labour	5 490 000	151	
			Liberal	2 930 000	40	1 217 000 (11.2%)

APPENDIX 1 (*contd*)

Gen. Election Date	Party	Prime Minister	Voting Party	Number	Seats	Unemployment
1929 May	Labour	Ramsey MacDonald	Conservative	8 660 000	260	
			Labour	8 390 000	288	
			Liberal	5 310 000	59	
1931 November	National	Ramsey MacDonald	Cons (Nat)	13 129 000	521	2 630 000 (21.5%)
			Labour	6 650 000	52	
			Liberal	1 403 000	33	2 521 000 (21.3%)
1935 November	National	Stanley Baldwin	Cons (Nat)	11 810 000	432	2 290 000 (18.7%)
	Conservative	Neville Chamberlain (1937)	Labour	8 325 000	154	1 810 000 (14.8%)
	Coalition	Winston Churchill (1940)	Liberal	1 422 000	20	
1945 July	Labour	Clement Attlee	Conservative	9 988 000	213	2.50%
			Labour	11 995 000	393	
			Liberal	2 248 000	12	
			Other	854 000	22	

APPENDIX 1 (*contd*)

Gen. Election *Date*	Party	Prime Minister	Voting *Party*	*Number*	*Seats*	Unemployment
1950 March	Labour	Clement Attlee	Conservative	12 503 000	298	2.50%
			Labour	13 267 000	315	
			Liberal	2 622 000	9	
			Other	382 000	3	
1951 October	Conservative	Winston Churchill	Conservative	13 718 000	321	2.50%
			Labour	13 949 000	295	
			Liberal	731 000	6	
			Other	Not known	3	
1955 May	Conservative	Sir Anthony Eden	Conservative	13 287 000	344	2.50%
			Labour	12 405 000	277	
			Liberal	722 400	6	
			Other	Not known	3	
1959 October	Conservative	Harold Macmillan Sir Alec Douglas-Home (1963)	Conservative	13 750 000	365	2.50%
			Labour	12 215 000	258	
			Liberal	1 639 000	6	
			Other	Not known	1	

APPENDIX 1 *contd*

Gen. Election Date	Party	Prime Minister	Voting Party	Number	Seats	Unemployment
1964 October	Labour	Harold Wilson	Labour	12 206 000	317	2.50%
			Conservative	12 001 000	304	
			Liberal	3 093 000	9	
1966 March	Labour	Harold Wilson	Labour	13 065 000	363	2.50%
			Conservative	12 179 000	253	
			Liberal	2 328 000	12	
			Other	Not known	2	
1970 June	Conservative	Edward Heath	Conservative	13 145 000	330	3.20%
			Labour	12 179 000	287	
			Liberal	2 117 000	6	
			Other	906 000	7	
1974 February	Labour	Harold Wilson	Labour	11 639 000	301	3.20%
			Conservative	11 869 000	297	
			Liberal	6 063 000	14	
			Other	804 000	23	

APPENDIX 1 (*contd*)

Gen. Election Date	Party	Prime Minister	Voting Party	Number	Seats	Unemployment
1974 October	Labour	Harold Wilson	Labour	11 457 000	319	6.00%
		James Callaghan	Conservative	10 465 000	277	
		(1976)	Liberal	5 347 000	13	
			Other	804 000	26	
1979 May	Conservative	Margaret Thatcher	Conservative	13 698 000	339	6.40%
			Labour	11 523 000	269	
			Liberal	4 314 000	11	
			Other	1 678 000	16	12.40%
1983 June	Conservative	Margaret Thatcher	Conservative	13 012 000	397	11.70%
			Labour	8 457 000	209	
			Alliance	7 781 000	23	
			Other	1 222 000	21	10.30%
1987 June	Conservative	Margaret Thatcher	Conservative	13 736 000	376	9.10%
			Labour	10 030 000	229	
			Alliance	7 341 000	22	
			Other	1 270 000	23	8.70%

APPENDIX 1 (*contd*)

Gen. Election Date	Party	Prime Minister	Voting Party	Number	Seats	Unemployment
1992 April	Conservative	John Major	Conservative	14 093 000	336	9.10%
			Labour	11 560 000	271	
			Lib Dem	5 999 000	20	
			Other	1 961 000	24	7.20%
1997 May	New Labour	Tony Blair	Labour	13 518 000	418	7.00%
			Conservative	9 601 000	165	
			Lib Dem	5 243 000	46	
			Other	2 924 000	30	

APPENDIX 2

US Presidents

1901–1909	Theodore Roosevelt
1909–1913	William Howard Taft
1913–1921	Woodrow Wilson
1921–1923	Warren G Harding
1923–1929	Calvin Coolidge
1929–1933	Herbert G Hoover
1933–1945	Franklin D Roosevelt
1945–1953	Harry S Truman
1953–1961	Dwight D Eisenhower
1961–1963	John F Kennedy
1963–1969	Lyndon B Johnson
1969–1974	Richard M Nixon
1974–1977	Gerald R Ford
1977–1981	James E Carter
1981–1989	Ronald W Reagan
1989–1993	George HW Bush
1993–2001	William J Clinton

6. What has Influenced Epidemiological Public Health Research?

Our aim in the earlier chapters of this book has been to analyse the research output in EPHR since the end of World War I. There have been very significant improvements both in the health of the population and in the organisation and delivery of health services in this period. We have tried to identify the most important research in the United Kingdom and the United States that may have contributed to these developments.

Role of Epidemiology

In the nineteenth century, epidemiology and public health research was largely concerned with the investigation of the major infections and hazards to which the population was exposed – for example, cholera, overcrowding, poor sanitation – and the exposure of specific groups to serious environmental hazards – for example, child chimney sweeps who developed scrotal cancers. It was in both our countries a highly "political" subject and its practitioners were, in general, missionaries intent on improving the health of the population.

In the twentieth century the discipline, its practitioners and the milieu had changed. There was a real improvement in health and life conditions but many problems remained. Between 1919 and 1939 there was a great deal of unemployment, poverty and environmental degradation. Although researchers in EPHR were motivated to improve the health of the population, they were equally, if not more, concerned with an increase in scientific knowledge and, in both the UK and US, were somewhat distant from those involved in the implementation of research findings.

After 1945, although there was still a major effort to determine the aetiology of specific conditions and their control, public health practitioners became much more closely involved in efficacy and effectiveness research in medicine more generally, in contrast to the previous focus on immunising agents or vaccines used in the control of infectious disease. Part of the reason for this may have been the impetus given to this type of research by the development of the applicability of randomised controlled trials by Bradford Hill and others, and the realisation that this technique could be used in the assessment not only of individual drugs but also of services and organisational structures. This was accompanied by the application of epidemiological methods and designs to health services research.

Interest in the Subject

Policy-makers involved in health, environmental and social issues have always had an interest in EPHR. It is difficult to judge whether there has been any change in this relationship. It is true, however, that media interest in the findings of EPHR has increased considerably over time – it is now rare not to find mention of some EPHR finding in a newspaper, magazine, or TV programme. Science editors have become reasonably knowledgeable in their use of EPHR findings although there remains great confusion about the use of absolute and relative risk, and more caution is needed in the interpretation of ecological type and case-control studies and the difference between pragmatic and experimental investigations. Media interest has been encouraged by some researchers in their quest for fame and funds.

With the rapid dissemination of some epidemiological risk findings to the public, problems have arisen because there has been no opportunity for confirmation or refutation, and because some of the caveats of interpretation understood and used by trained professionals are misunderstood or neglected by the media and propagandists in the interests of getting a "good story".

There has been increasing interest in EPHR findings among lawyers and industrialists. In the former, EPHR is increasingly being used in toxic tort cases and in environmental regulation and risk assessment. Courts have begun to use epidemiological evidence in their rulings and one of us (LG) has even become involved in running courses for judges to improve their understanding of the field. This has encouraged industry to sponsor and fund EPHR studies and training and has contributed to the growth, particularly in the US, of private, for profit, epidemiological and consulting research, particularly in environmental and pharmaco-epidemiology.

Changes in Practice

EPHR has always been multidisciplinary and there has always been some degree of rivalry between those with a medical qualification and those without, well exemplified by the attitudes to and between Chadwick (a layman) and John Simon (a surgeon) in the nineteenth century. Perhaps one of the most productive and able researchers in the twentieth century was Austin Bradford Hill, not a doctor but a medical statistician. It is noteworthy, however, that in all his EPHR, he worked closely with doctors and his understanding of the biological processes and background was always equal to and sometimes better than that of the doctors with whom he collaborated.

A marked change in EPHR has been a shift in emphasis and type of research done. Epidemiology has become highly statistical and there has been a shift from emphasis on research, designed to answer biologically important and meaningful questions with the planned collection of data, to reliance on statistical methods (to correct for variability and biases) and large databases collected for routine administrative purposes. Concern with the reliability and validity of information used in EPHR has been replaced with reliance on sophisticated statistical methods and modelling, sometimes with sensitivity analyses. This change in approach has resulted in numerous publications – for example, Beaglehole and Bonita,[1] Susser,[2] Danish Symposium[3] – questioning the direction of our subject and its relevance to health policy. There are now many epidemiologists, some in senior positions, who have never undertaken any field studies or examined individuals.

At the beginning of the twentieth century, EPHR was largely concerned with the control and prevention of infectious diseases. This has changed gradually to a greater focus on chronic diseases and the last 35 years have shown a very marked growth of interest in health services research. With the increase in complexity as well as the effectiveness of health services, epidemiological approaches have been increasingly used both in the evaluation of services and techniques and in resource allocation, planning and management.

A major change has been the shift from small-scale studies to investigations based on large databases – not always designed for EPHR. The ability to handle large databases, using computing techniques, has certainly eased the problems of undertaking large studies on populations over long periods of time. Studies such as the British doctors' study on smoking and lung cancer by Hill and Doll on about 50 000 individuals, and the study by Cuyler Hammond on over one million Cancer Society volunteers on the same problem, were exceptional 40 years ago. Now they are commonplace.

This has been accompanied by the development of many large multicentre studies, whether randomised controlled trials, case-control studies or cohort studies. The best early example of these was the trial of poliomyelitis immunisation by Francis and his colleagues (March of Dimes)[4] but a recent example is the prevention and treatment of coronary heart disease with aspirin.[5]

The use of EPHR in such large studies on diverse topics, such as the delivery of health and social services as well as disease control, has been accompanied by an increase in concern with ethical issues in this form of research.

Dissemination of Research Findings

With the increase in the amount of research, there has been a rise in the number of publications. In the UK, for example, before 1939 there was only one specific journal in the field (the *Journal of Hygiene*), but there are now at least two more – the *Journal of Epidemiology and Community Health* and the *Journal of Public Health Medicine*. Many others, such as *Social Science and Medicine*, devote many pages in each issue to the subject. In the US, the *American Journal of Hygiene* (now *Epidemiology*) has been joined by the *Annals of Epidemiology*, the *Journal of Clinical Epidemiology* and other related journals. The number of books published has also expanded considerably. This increase in publications has been accompanied by the creation of a number of scientific societies – for example, the Society of Social Medicine, the Society of Epidemiologic Research, American Epidemiological Society. International bodies, in particular the International Epidemiological Association with the *International Journal of Epidemiology*, have served as a stimulus to the creation of many regional and national associations, often with their own journal.

The creation of these societies and publications has been linked to an increase in the national, regional and international conferences, symposia and seminars at which research findings are presented and discussed. Many general (and specialty) medical journals also include epidemiological papers, usually limited to those relevant to the particular field, and also include the discipline in their national and international meetings.

Finance

In both the US and UK, expenditure on EPHR has fluctuated over time. In general, expenditure on EPHR has increased markedly in both countries, both relatively and absolutely. It is difficult to be at all accurate on how much is spent in either country, whether by individual agency or research council, because a system for recording such expenditure classified as EPHR does not exist. Thus, for example, research may be classified under the heading of heart disease rather than the epidemiology of heart disease. Universities, the major site of most EPHR, do not classify their expenditure under subject headings either. Few, nonetheless, would argue that the total amount of resources, whether measured in number of researchers or in actual expenditure, has increased several fold. This is well demonstrated by the increase in number of public health posts in the UK and is mirrored by NIH figures on total expenditure. Although in the UK there were several years, between 1982 and 1996, when the resources for EPHR research were reduced, the general trend has been to increase the resources available. In the US there has been a major increase in NIH funding since 1945, although the rate of increase from year to year has varied.

Sources of Funding
In both countries there are three main categories of funder: university funding, government agencies and voluntary agencies. Industry, particularly the pharmaceutical firms, also fund specific studies, largely related to their products.

Location
In the United Kingdom before the World War I, EPHR was largely conducted in universities, medical schools, and local authority departments. With the foundation of the Medical Research Council, some epidemiologists began to be based in MRC establishments. This was developed after World War II by the creation of a number of epidemiological and social medicine research units as discussed in chapter 4.[6] The Ministry of Health began to create a number of research units in 1968. In 1923 the London School of Hygiene was founded and this has continued to be the only University School of Public Health.

In the United States, by contrast, there has been since the eighteenth century the US Public Health Service (USPHS), formerly the Marine Hospital Service. Since the end of the World War II, the National Institutes of Health have taken on many of the research roles of the USPHS (of which they are a part). Not only does NIH provide funds for training and research on public health, but each of the categorical institutes – for example, Heart, Cancer, Mental Health – includes an identifiable research branch/laboratory and they also fund research units in universities.

The main locus of EPHR in the US has been the Schools of Public Health or Hygiene which have increased in both number and size since the creation of the School at Johns Hopkins in 1912. A major change has been the increase in the number of departments of epidemiology and epidemiologists in medical schools in the past 20 years, particularly in the last decade. This has been linked to an increase in the teaching of epidemiology to medical students and in the amount of EPHR in schools of medicine. The use of biomarkers in epidemiology has, perhaps, served as a bridge to schools of medicine and practising clinicians.

Personnel

With the growth in resources there has been a concomitant increase in the number of active researchers. In the early years most senior researchers – with the notable exceptions of Bradford Hill, Sydenstricker, Yerushalmy, Pearl and others – were medically qualified. The situation has changed. In the past 30 years there has been a very marked increase in the number of non-medically qualified researchers involved. These have included medical statisticians, social scientists, psychologists, geographers, economists, biologists and representatives of many other disciplines including politics.

Differential pay scales between those working in a medical institution and those in a non-medical one have had an influence. More detrimental to the field has been the higher pay of medically qualified persons compared to those without such a qualification within an individual department. The high earnings of medical practitioners who care for patients, compared to those who do not, have had a major impact on the recruitment and retention of such people in EPHR in the US. In the UK the major difference in medical earnings is between those who practise privately and those who do not. The differential is thus less of a problem since most of the doctors choosing to do EPHR do not undertake private practice. There are potential difficulties in the UK in the future. The gap between researchers in academia and those in commerce or in the services is widening. Current attitudes and media interest may also widen the differences in pay between those in glamourised acute specialties in contrast to those in less obviously glamorous fields such as public health, creating similar differentials to those current in the US.

In both the UK and the US, recognition of "specialist" qualification as an epidemiologist has been relatively recent. In the UK, the founding of the Faculty of Community Medicine in 1972 (now the Faculty of Public Health Medicine) enabled medical academics to be included and provided with appropriate training and certification of competence. For those doing solely academic research, this has produced a number of difficulties which, however, could be overcome, and have been discussed in detail elsewhere. More difficult has been the "accreditation" of non-medical researchers – but this too has begun to be tackled in recent years. In the US, there was a lack of federal recognition for epidemiology – epidemiologists working in federal institutions have to be labelled as statisticians. This has been solved in 1979 with the foundation of the American College of Epidemiology.

Conditions Required to Optimise EPHR

EPHR is undertaken in many types of institution. For effective, productive research it is essential that researchers work in a clearly identifiable unit or department. These are usually located in a University, Medical School, School of Public Health or other type of national, regional or local health institution – for example, National Institutes of Health, MRC Unit or Centre, Institute of Public Health, within a Regional or Local Health Board or Authority. It is crucial that the unit or department has close links with other research or academic units concerned with health in order to facilitate the identification of appropriate questions to research as well as to benefit from the knowledge, experience, facilities and equipment available in related fields of expertise. Thus units or departments located, for example, in a purely managerial setting such as a Ministry or in a commercial or free-standing private company are unlikely to be very productive in EPHR.

Over the time examined, there has been a steady growth in the facilities and institutions involved in EPHR in both countries. As described, there are differences between the UK and the US. In the UK, EPHR is largely based in universities and MRC units. In the US, it is also based within universities and the NIH, although there are several commercial research units starting to appear. In the US the involvement of medical schools is relatively recent and most output and training has been in Schools of Public Health, institutions of enviable size when compared to the one solitary School in London.

Productivity of EPHR

There are a series of factors or conditions which enable researchers to be productive in EPHR. The most important in our view can be summarised under the following headings.

Effective Recruitment

Before 1939 most EPHR researchers in the UK received no formal training in research or in the field. Training in medical statistics was absent until the foundation of the London School of Hygiene. Investigators such as Major Greenwood with both a medical qualification and statistical expertise were extremely rare. Public Health Medical Officers required a Diploma in Public Health (DPH), and training for this was provided in a variety of Schools, as described by Fee and Acheson.[6] A few of these developed research, often from a service base – for example, M'Gonigle. The most common background of researchers was, however, in the laboratory disciplines such as bacteriology (microbiology) or biochemistry. To undertake research in the UK pre-1939 was not a lucrative proposition – many researchers had private means. Nonetheless some very able individuals were active.

In the US the situation was similar except that there was a national body, the US Public Health Service, which had as one of its missions undertaking and supporting EPHR – in contrast to the UK where no such national body existed.

After 1945 there was a change in the UK. A number of very able and charismatic individuals became interested in the field – among them Cochrane, Doll, Morris, McKeown, Reid and Stewart. Obviously, their experiences both before and during the war stimulated them in devising appropriate important investigations in its aftermath. Reid, for example, became involved in studies of bomber pilot fatigue and stress.

They recruited a number of talented individuals to work with them – Backett, Brotherston, Knowelden, Last, Pemberton. There was thus a relatively small core of charismatic researchers in EPHR, mostly self-taught. The DPH courses continued. There was, however, a major problem in the recruitment of medically qualified individuals into the field. In the creation of the National Health Service, public health was separated from clinical services. Public health doctors worked for local authorities and their pay scale was different from and lower than that applying to clinicians.[7] Epidemiologists in academic institutions were not considered to be clinicians and so were paid on a lower salary scale. It was only the creation of academic departments in medical schools and universities, independent of service public health, that enabled the salaries of medically qualified teachers in these departments to be linked to those of other clinical teachers. The clear recognition that public health and epidemiology teaching was linked to clinical medicine also helped. The creation of the Faculty of Community Medicine (Public Health) and the change in structure of the organisation of the NHS which brought public health from local authority to NHS jurisdiction were the final acts which ensured that the pay of EPHR researchers was similar to that of other medical researchers.

Ensuring comparable pay did help recruitment to the specialty. There were, however, other obstacles. Until 1972 the only recognised courses for public health were the DPH at the London School of Hygiene and various other UK universities.[6] This diploma was not designed for those wishing to do research. There were a number of short courses at the London School of Hygiene in epidemiology and medical statistics which provided a grounding in the field. But most researchers learnt on the job without much formal training.

In the US, the situation was a little better. The courses for the Master of Public Health (MPH) and for Doctorates at the Schools of Public Health were more suited to provide research background and training.

The UK MRC recognised this deficit in the early 1960s and a number of future senior academics were encouraged, and funded, to spend time in academic institutions in the USA.

For the period up to 1975 the dearth of places to train in EPHR in the UK was very marked. Only one or two departments recognised the need to provide properly supervised training in EPHR.

Since 1975 the situation has changed markedly so that there are not only recognised courses and qualifications but also funding for research fellowships from a variety of sources. This has had an effect on recruitment of researchers in both countries. The discipline-mix of researchers, however, has changed, with a far higher proportion of non-medically qualified individuals. This is partly because of the differences between the earnings of those with a medical degree who have clinical duties or private practice and those in research, but also because institutions find it cheaper to hire non-medical researchers.

Quality of Field Work

Although many findings of importance in EPHR are based on analysis and evaluation of data, we consider it crucial that future researchers have experience of collecting such data "in the field". Only by practical experience of what some call "shoe leather epidemiology" can future researchers learn of the relevance and validity of data used in EPHR. This should involve both the design and the administration of surveys and investigations so as to make the future researcher aware of the complexities involved in field work. The trend toward research based largely on large data sets – often collected for other purposes – is detrimental to the advances and credibility of EPHR.

Freedom of Publication

The opportunities for publication and dissemination of research results have improved greatly in the past 30 years. It is important for all EPHR to ensure that researchers are not prevented or inhibited from publishing their findings, even if they make uncomfortable reading for the commissioners of research.

For all EPHR it is absolutely crucial that researchers are free to publish their views. Findings are frequently contrary to government industrial and commercial policies and interests, which is why researchers must remain independent of political and managerial structures. Since EPHR is concerned with improving the health of populations it is essential that populations learn about, and trust, its findings – this is difficult for some managers and politicians to accept. An example in 1968 was the experience of the author (WWH) in putting forward a scheme of research on what, at that time, was known as "Best Buy Hospitals". At the initial meeting with officials, a senior Health Ministry Medical Officer queried the proposal, saying, "but what if it does not support our policy?". It took about six months of internal discussion within the Ministry to accept that the purpose of the research was to question its policy and evaluate it. This example has been repeated many times – for example, evidence to House of Lords Select Committee.[8]

Continuing Questions

EPHR is an applied topic. It is, therefore, necessary that research questions address real problems and not just theoretical possibilities. The variety of relevant questions is vast and researchers need to be selective in what is tackled. It helps to be in touch with those responsible for the delivery of services, to learn of their questions and problems. Close links to service delivery and implementation are to be welcomed and encouraged.

Access to Services and Populations

Almost all EPHR is carried out on defined population groups or on patients. It is thus necessary that researchers have easy access to services and populations – obviously this is easier if there are close links. An advantage of EPHR within a medical school sited in a hospital is the natural linkage between public health and clinical service – meeting the responsible individuals as well as having easy access to patient groups/laboratories, etc. A disadvantage is that these locations are rarely suitable for non-medical basic disciplines such as sociology, economics and so on.

Discipline

EPHR is and must be very much an interdisciplinary activity. It is rare that any one individual, or one discipline, can encompass all the facets of the problem under investigation. Epidemiologists need to work with statisticians, health economists, sociologists, social psychologists, geographers, and anthropologists, to name but some of the disciplines involved. Further access is needed to laboratories – microbiological, biochemical and toxicological – in order to investigate some of the questions. Schools of Public Health are more welcoming institutions than medical schools for some of these varying disciplines. Thus it is advantageous for EPHR to be located in such institutions rather than in purely medical ones. The important thing to recognise is that no locus is ideal; each has its advantages and disadvantages.

Data Protection

All EPHR is dependent on information collected on either well populations or patients. Often some of this data will have been collected in the past and be present in medical or other records. Although researchers have always recognised the need for confidentiality of information collected and have included safeguards in their protocols, new obstacles have arisen. Data protection laws in European countries and the US have been enacted, largely in response to population fears and the advent of far easier data manipulation and storage, which do place obstacles in the way of EPHR. Medical information collected in the past on an individual, for example, may not be released to a researcher unless permission is given by the individual concerned. This certainly raises serious issues for EPHR, – and will need to be resolved, since otherwise much vital retrospective research will become impossible.

Conclusion

In this chapter we have described some of the conditions necessary for the conduct of EPHR and trends over time which may have influenced the work carried out. We have also aimed to highlight some important issues that need to be tackled to ensure the continuation of effective EPHR on both sides of the Atlantic into the twenty-first century.

REFERENCES

1 Beaglehole R, Bonita R. (1997) *Public Health at the Crossroads*. Cambridge: Cambridge University Press.

2 Susser M, Susser E. (1996) Choosing a future for epidemiology. *American Journal of Public Health*, 86: 668–673; 674–678.

3 The First Panum Lecture in Copenhagen. (1999) Saracci R, Wall S, Adami HO, et al. *International Journal of Epidemiology*, 25: S996–S1024.

4 Francis I, Napier RB, Voight FM. (1955) Evaluation of 1954 field trials of poliomyelitis vaccine. *American Journal of Public Health*, 45: 5.

5 Elwood PC, Cochrane AL, Brown ML, et al. (1974) A randomised, controlled trial of acetylsalicylic acid in the secondary prevention of mortality from myocardial infarction. *British Medical Journal*, 1: 436–440.

6 Fee E, Acheson RM (Eds). (1991) *A History of Education in Public Health*. Oxford: Oxford University Press.

7 Holland WW, Stewart S. (1998) *Public Health: The Vision and the Challenge*. London: Nuffield Trust.

8 Select Committee on Science and Technology. (1988) *Priorities in Medical Research*. House of Lords, Paper 54-I, London: HMSO.

7. Conclusion

We have tried in this book to describe the major research undertaken in the United Kingdom and the United States in epidemiological public health research (EPHR), to illuminate health policy in our two countries since the end of World War I. There have been major improvements in health over these eight decades and the research carried out has undoubtedly contributed to this. We have also described the most important structures involved in this research and attempted to analyse the political and social changes which have taken place. The bibliography for this chapter is short since we have not quoted again most of the many references cited earlier in the book.

In reviewing the research output overall, we can see that much more EPHR has been carried out in recent years than at the beginning of the period. Obviously the amount of research possible is influenced greatly by the amount of resource – both human and material – available. The US is a much bigger country and the amount expended on research is greater than in the UK. Braun[1] has described the arrangements for the support for public health research in the two countries, and illustrates the quantitative differences in the fiscal provisions. We have tried to describe the differences, over time, in the arrangements for research, as well as the research done.

There have been major changes in the balance of EPHR problems investigated. Between the World Wars most such research was concerned with infectious diseases and with nutrition. There were beginnings of a greater concentration on quantitative and experimental rather than anecdotal work but the development of methods for the investigation of disease in populations was dominated by an approach developed in laboratories. After World War II, the types of research shifted coincidentally with the change in the causes of disease. Although infectious diseases were still important, the advent of effective methods of treatment with antibiotics, in particular, meant that these conditions became less central as a cause of mortality – and thus of lesser interest to researchers. At the same time, advances in microbiological knowledge led to the development of effective immunising agents – for example for polio, measles and whooping cough – and most importantly, improvements in nutrition and hygiene had a major impact in reducing the burden of illness from these conditions.

The main causes of ill health in both countries were now the chronic diseases such as cancer, cardiovascular and respiratory diseases, mental illness and rheumatic conditions. To investigate these, epidemiological methods required change and development, and methods of inquiry needed to be adapted to the investigation of conditions with a far longer natural history than, for example, diarrhoea or pneumonia. In addition, advances in clinical methods of treatment and care enabled health services to have a very marked effect on both quality of life and outcome. These thus became worthy objects of investigation. Prevention now also entailed far more complex procedures than, for example, a new vaccine or a clean water supply.

In the immediate past 15 years or so there has been a further shift in research interests. With the emergence of HIV/AIDS there has been a renewal of interest in infectious disease. Advances in molecular biology and genetics have also stimulated a greater interest in laboratory methods in public health research. The advances in knowledge and research in the period 1945–1975 of the major factors concerned with the aetiology of common conditions such as coronary heart disease, cancer of the lung, and chronic respiratory disease have meant that EPHR has changed. Since the "plums" have been gathered, much of the research has tended to be repetitive and concerned with clarifying detail. Disappointingly little new research has been initiated on other chronic conditions, such as mental illness or locomotor injuries, which have a low profile. This may be, of course, because of the greater difficulties of disentangling or identifying aetiological factors in these conditions. The suspicion remains, however, that this lack of interest is the result both of the public image of these mundane conditions and of the imperative to publish definitive findings – much easier in a well-defined field than in a new area.

We subdivided the period for review into three different segments. These were arbitrary but coincided, to some extent, with natural socio-political end-points: 1919–1939, 1945–1975, 1975–1999. Each segment was approximately 25 years long.

1919–1939

Between 1919 and 1939 research in the US appeared to be of higher quality and more relevant to the needs of the population, in both the short- and long-term, than in the UK. Perhaps the best illustration of this is provided by research on infectious disease, arguably the most common health problem at that time. In the UK a very great deal of effort was expended on artificial experiments of transmission of infection in mouse colonies by Topley and his colleagues over many years. Although these studies consumed a large proportion of the expenditure of the MRC on EPHR, they were not fruitful in the control of infectious disease.[2] By contrast, the work of Pearl and Wade Hampton Frost, in the US at this time, remains central to our understanding of the spread of diseases such as measles and typhoid and continues to be used in our control strategies for infections.

Although the influenza virus was isolated by Andrewes and his colleagues at Mill Hill, the number of outstanding studies on the prevention and control of infectious conditions, such as poliomyelitis, whooping cough and measles, was not equivalent to studies in the United States by Paul, Francis or others. There were important investigations on streptococcal infections – for example, by Colebrook on puerperal fever in the UK, equivalent to those by Rammelkamp and his colleagues in the US in advancing our knowledge of these infections.

Neglect of diphtheria immunisation in the UK (shown to be effective in US and Canadian studies by 1930) led to some 20 000 avoidable deaths before universal immunisation was introduced in 1941.[5]

Tuberculosis is another example where UK research lagged behind US. Although the initial impetus to the formation of the Medical Research Committee (later Medical Research Council) in 1913 was tuberculosis, Bryden[2] noted lack of interest after 1919 by the Council in this disease, in spite of the immense burden of this condition on the British population, until the appointment of Dr D'Arcy Hart in the late 1930s. This is perhaps best illustrated by the lack of involvement of British workers in the development of effective control measures for TB until after World War II,[2] and contrasts with the work of Carol Palmer and others in the US.

These judgments are not intended to denigrate the work of individual practitioners or researchers such as Pickles, a general practitioner in Wensleydale, who developed valuable knowledge of the natural history of infections in general practice, or Cruickshank on the aerial spread of streptococcal infections, but to highlight the relative dearth of important contributions in the UK compared to the US.

Research into occupational and industrial factors was largely descriptive in both the UK and the US. This period saw the beginning of interest into the specific effects of hazards such as coal mining, working in cotton mills and the effects of exposure to lead, but, in general, there were few really good epidemiological investigations in this field in either country.

With the advances in knowledge of biochemistry and the visible effects of poverty on the nutritional status of the population, it is not surprising that there were many examples of research on nutrition or nutritional factors in both countries. This era saw an explosion of interest in the role of vitamins and other accessory factors, as well as the total consumption of nutrients, on health. Although there were many important studies by a variety of British workers such as Chick, the Mellanbys, McCarrison, and in later years, Widdowson and McCance, only Boyd Orr and M'Gonigle in the UK tackled the problems of nutrition from a satisfactory population perspective. Boyd Orr, in his surveys of the diet of samples of the British population linked to examination of their physical and medical status, and bolstered by animal experiments, showed the variations in diet between different social groups and the beneficial effects of a good diet on health and growth. His studies underpinned food policy (rationing) during World War II and ensured that the population of Britain never starved but in fact improved in health, in spite of the U-boat blockade and restriction of food supplies.

M'Gonigle's studies on the health of the poor in Stockton-on-Tees demonstrated the link between poverty and food intake. It is surprising, in view of the unemployment and poverty of a large proportion of the UK population, that so few good studies were carried out. By contrast, the studies by Goldberger and his colleagues in the Southern US on the importance of nutritional deficiencies in the aetiology of pellagra were very influential in improving the diets of prisoners and poor black people and are still recognised as models of epidemiological investigation.

Although there were many other reasonable EPHR investigations in the UK during this period which are described in chapter 2, they do not match the number or quality of studies done in the US. Thus the development of the population laboratory in Hagerstown in 1922 by Sydenstricker and the work on the provision of health care by Falk are but two examples of outstanding research.

Underlying this, however, was the US commitment to investigate and improve the health of those at greatest disadvantage – as clearly communicated in the objectives of the USPHS.

The enormous growth in American scientific research in general, after the beginning of the twentieth century, in comparison with other countries, has been documented.[3]

1945–1975

The first 20 years after the end of World War II were probably the golden years of EPHR in the UK. Although the number of researchers involved was not large, the renown of those such as Bradford Hill, Cochrane, Doll, McKeown, Reid, Stewart, and many others is still remembered. These individuals can be considered to have made outstanding contributions both to the development of methods and to knowledge on aetiology and how to control the most important hazards to health. Our debt to them is immense.

Although many contributions were made to infectious disease control in the UK at this time, they were probably not as significant as those made in the US. Examples of this are the contrast between the studies on poliomyelitis and its prevention, acute respiratory infections and the development and testing of appropriate vaccines, the prevention and control of tuberculosis, and the establishment of a national system of surveillance at the Centre for Disease Control (CDC) which later was copied in the UK (CDSC).

Perhaps the most striking achievement in the UK at this time was in the development of field methods for the investigation of chronic diseases through the use of questionnaires and other reliable methods of measuring physiological and pathological characteristics in defined population groups. This was linked to the development of methods by which defined population groups, geographic or occupational, could be exploited to answer a wide variety of questions relating to the aetiology and prevention of chronic conditions. This was combined with the rigorous assessment of sources of variability and bias in the conduct of these investigations, enabling more reliable conclusions to be drawn.

Although similar developments were occurring in the United States – for instance, by the continuing studies in Hagerstown, the use of Tecumseh,

Michigan in a number of studies of coronary heart disease, Alameda County and many other sites – it is usually acknowledged that the UK studies were slightly superior. A good example is the study of lung cancer. The initial case-control studies showing the association of lung cancer and smoking cigarettes, by Hill and Doll, Wynder and Graham and Levin, were published almost simultaneously. Although Hammond and Horn mounted a very interesting prospective study in Cancer Society volunteers and Dorn in Veterans, Hill and Doll's prospective study in medical practitioners is the only one to have continued for more than 40 years and was the first to demonstrate reliably that stopping smoking was effective in reducing the risk of developing lung cancer – an extremely important public health message.

It is difficult to judge the relative merits of studies of the epidemiology of coronary heart disease. In the USA the studies started by Dawber and Kannel in Framingham continued to provide important and relevant information, even though the original design was flawed because of the relatively low response rate and reliance, initially, on clinical observations without regard for the problems of observer variability. The work by Breslow, Epstein, Keys and many others also made fundamental contributions. On the other hand, the work of Morris, Rose, Reid and others was equally fundamental – from a purely academic view it yielded crucial findings with a parsimonious use of resources and was probably sounder and more reliable methodologically.

There are many other examples where studies were done in both countries, all contributing to our knowledge of respiratory disease, cancer, psychiatry, health services and philosophy but the general impression that UK research was slightly more advanced and better than that of the US in this period remains.

1975–1999
In the final period of our survey, it is more difficult to reach clear conclusions. We believe, looking at published research and taking into account the vastly different level of resource available for research in the two countries, that the quality of US research was maintained, and perhaps improved, while that in the UK began to decline. Judgments are difficult because, as we have already said, most of the "plums" had already been picked, so that much of the enquiry in both countries investigated small, detailed areas rather than big pictures. In the field of infectious disease, US predominance continued to be clear – as exemplified

by US work on HIV/AIDS. As a contrast, the British studies on BSE/ Creutzfeldt-Jakob were flawed (see annexe 2).

These comparisons demonstrate that there were differences in the output of EPHR in our two countries in the last century. In this conclusion it is worth summarising both the changes which have occurred in the organisation and the type of research done during this period, as well as some of the factors which we consider to be important in the promotion of productive EPHR. Finally, we will attempt to relate these to the organisation and conditions which have been described.

Structure and Resources

Although there are differences in the organisation of research and medical/ health education between the UK and the US, there are many similarities. In the US the major public (federal) institution both funding and supporting EPHR is the National Institutes of Health. In the UK, the MRC serves the same function. There was, however, a major difference of focus between them at least until after World War II. The US Public Health Service, founded in 1789, originally as the Marine Hospital Service, was specifically created "for the temporary relief and maintenance of sick or disabled seamen".[2] In 1889 it was renamed the US Public Health Service with a specific remit "to focus on the poor, the exploited and the ill represented". In 1891 it opened a Hygiene Laboratory on Staten Island to investigate the illnesses of seamen and immigrants but soon realised the wider potential of this institution and moved to Washington. The Laboratory served as a base for the development of preventive methods, including vaccines.

The commissioned corps of officers was charged with expansion of research and development of disease control (acute and chronic) programmes. Thus it is not surprising that many of the eminent researchers between the wars – such as Goldberger, Wade Hampton Frost and Sydenstricker – were employed by the USPHS. The USPHS was also responsible for initiating the establishment in Hagerstown of a "population laboratory". Almost all the major efforts to investigate or control common conditions such as tuberculosis or venereal diseases were initiated and funded through the USPHS, with the close involvement of both present and past members of the commissioned corps of officers. After 1938, the Hygiene Laboratory became the nascent National Institutes of Health (NIH). The role of NIH became much wider, while the USPHS officers became more concerned with disease control and administration than with research.

This institutional base for concern with both the discovery and the application of public health knowledge, in the period up to 1939, was lacking in the UK. The purpose of the MRC was certainly the discovery of knowledge but as we have noted, its relationships with those responsible for its application were not good. Furthermore, the fundamental ethos and charge of the USPHS was to improve the lot of the poor and ill and this was not the case with the MRC.

A further difference between the UK and the US in the period up to 1939 was the academic base for public health. In the UK, as already discussed, public health education and research was scattered; there were few major centres of expertise and only one School of Public Health, founded with the generosity of the American Rockefeller Foundation. By contrast there were several universities in the USA, led by Johns Hopkins, Harvard, Philadelphia and Columbia, with well endowed public health institutions. Many of the leaders of these were retired USPHS staff with expertise and interest in EPHR.

In the period 1945–1975 the problems tackled by EPHR were often more concerned with chronic disease – for example, cancer of the lung or coronary heart disease. Access to clinical bases and knowledge became important to investigate these. Until about 1985, Schools of Public Health were very separate from medical schools and had relatively little interest in clinical medicine. Thus the dearth of Schools of Public Health in the UK was no longer as important in providing a base for EPHR.

Before World War II, service public health in both the UK and the US was largely concerned with the control of disease through legislative and hygienic measures. As has been noted before,[5] few public health departments in the UK were interested in the development of research. In the USA, however, the USPHS had specific remits for the development of knowledge *and* the control of disease.

After 1945 major developments and expansion of NIH research facilities began. In the UK the MRC became very supportive of epidemiological research. Although the UK developed a national Public Health Laboratory Service (similar to the Centre for Disease Control, Atlanta) it was not until the late 1970s that it had a national capability for the investigation of outbreaks of communicable disease (CDSC) which was modelled on the US example.

Relations between EPHR and the service functions of public health remained separate in both countries until 1974. With the creation of the Faculty of Community Medicine (now public health medicine), academic and service practitioners followed a common pathway and relations became much closer. An American observer (P Fox, personal communication) commented that, from his experience, British researchers had much easier access to and involvement in central health service policy decisions than those in the US.

The expansion of research capacity in EPHR is similar in both countries after 1945 – although, of course, the resources available in the USA were much greater.

Before 1939 there was one other major difference between the two countries. The attitude of private, charitable institutions to EPHR was far more favourable in the US. The best example of this is the Rockefeller Foundation, which was responsible not only for the foundation of Johns Hopkins University School of Hygiene but also for the London School of Hygiene and other such schools and departments in Beijing and Rio de Janeiro. In the UK the involvement of charitable foundations in the support of EPHR did not really begin until the late 1930s with Lord Nuffield.

This American habit of massive support for EPHR from charitable foundations is not easy to explain but it has continued. It is true that great individual wealth was created in the USA from the end of the nineteenth century, whereas in the UK few individuals were able to amass huge fortunes on the scale of Rockefeller, Macy or Gates. There were (and are), however, individuals who are equally wealthy within the UK. But there is a fundamental difference. British wealth tends to be old money and passed on from generation to generation. It has been suggested that self-made men, who have themselves experienced poverty, are both more likely to support research intended to improve the lot of the poor but also to consider that their children should make their own way in life. This may explain, at least in part, the willingness of foundations created from new money to be more generous in the support of EPHR than those where the money was "older". There are, of course, exceptions. In the UK, Lord Nuffield, a self-made engineer, supported EPHR, and the Rowntree Foundation, Quaker in background, was active in the support of research on poverty from the nineteenth century onward.

Attitude of Professions

Relations between public health, epidemiology and clinical medicine have always been strained. Part of the problem is financial. Before the advent of the NHS in 1948, free clinical services were only available to the employed (insured) members of the population, or through charitable institutions – for example, voluntary hospitals – in the UK. Many public health departments, however, provided free services for some members of the population such as pregnant mothers, children and the elderly although this was opposed by some GPs concerned about loss of income.[5]

This was less of a problem in the United States where there was and still is no national insurance and where the competition for fees between the public and private sectors is much less marked because of the comparatively small size of the former.

In both countries, however, attitudes to population-based research is similar. Clinicians, who are concerned with the treatment of individuals, tend to be dismissive of population-based research where findings apply to groups rather than individuals. After the major advances in hygiene of the nineteenth century, the benefits of these tended to be accepted by both doctors and others involved in health policy. There was little support for EPHR, especially in the UK, until after the end of World War II. Most epidemiologists and public health workers were considered to be left-wing – not acceptable to the Establishment, which included the leaders of medicine. This attitude was confirmed by the participation of some of the future leaders of epidemiology, such as Cochrane, as recruits to the International Brigade in Spain. Many others were proponents of the introduction of a National Health Service – opposed by the majority of the medical profession.

This conservative attitude of the medical profession to EPHR mimicked the general attitude of society, as described above. World War II demonstrated the need for solidarity, and opinions slowly began to change in the UK as EPHR became more accepted – and supported.

The attitudes and behaviour of the medical profession are more important in the UK than in the US. In the latter, the presence of established, powerful Schools of Public Health and the existence of a national body (USPHS) provided far more support for EPHR than in the UK, where there was only one powerful academic focus, the London School of Hygiene. Attitudes towards research, in general, were far more positive in the US than the UK in the period 1919–1939.

Since 1945 the situation has changed. In both the US and UK the relevance of epidemiology to individual practice has been generally accepted. The success of public health measures, such as immunisation, has demonstrated the benefits. With the realisation that advances in medicine can only occur as a result of research, the support of EPHR has increased in both countries.

In recent years the practice of medicine has become far less authoritarian and more based on evaluated findings. This has led to concern with "evidence-based medicine" (EBM) and the acceptance that clinical practice must be based on facts rather opinions. Before 1960 there were relatively few proven facts on which to base practice or policy. Epidemiologists were in the forefront of developing critical analyses of practice and were questioning accepted wisdom. This did not make them popular. Now some consider that epidemiology is *the* basic science of clinical research and clinical medicine! Thus the situation for EPHR has changed in this respect. But, as we have said above, there are now other pitfalls and threats.

Politics and Society

The fundamental problem of EPHR over the years has been its relation to society and politics. The findings of EPHR have always had a "political –societal" dimension. The clearest example of this was the classical observation of John Snow on cholera in London which demonstrated the relationship between a contaminated water supply and mortality. This and other work indicating the importance of sanitary conditions threatened the income and power of some sections of society, for example, landlords, and was thus the subject of much political controversy and the cause of division among those concerned with reforms and improvements in living conditions and those threatened by such social improvements. In the twentieth century these divisions were still present, but were slightly different.

The two annexes to this chapter give stark specific examples of how politics and EPHR interact. The first contains a description of the conditions in the German

Democratic Republic (GDR) between its foundation and the fall of the Berlin Wall in 1989. The account has been written by an observer from West Berlin and is the result of both personal observations and discussions with colleagues active in the GDR before and after the fall of the Berlin Wall. It illustrates the problems of the ideological control of the type of research done as well as the way in which "factual" data was manipulated. Three examples are of particular note. Before the mid-1970s, when the price of imported oil was reasonable, research was done on the relationship of air pollution and respiratory disease. When the price of oil increased considerably, partly as the result of the Arab-Israeli War in 1973, brown coal production was increased enormously and most energy was generated from this source. The levels of air pollution increased considerably, evident by the palls of brown fumes and fog in the GDR. No further research on the health effects of this pollution was carried out.

The second example is research on social inequalities and associated effects of housing, etc. Since the State was based on the premise of social equality and new housing was a state priority, no work on this was permitted.

Finally, although epidemiological research was carried out on drugs and alcohol and their effects on health, the results of this were never allowed to be published!

By contrast, certain areas, such as immunisation, health surveillance, screening, occupational health and rehabilitation were the subject of much work. For some conditions such as tuberculosis, excellent services were provided.

Since the reunification of Germany, public health researchers from the GDR (with experience of working under the East and West regimes) have commented that, although there was now freedom to tackle all issues, resources for investigation of problems of particular concern to clinical practice and for pharmaceutical developments were much easier to obtain than, for example, resources for health services research.

It is of particular interest that, in spite of the ability of researchers in the East to be fully informed of research trends and findings in Western Europe and the USA, the State was able to constrain the ability to inquire into some "political-environmental" issues.

The second annexe describes a more recent episode in the UK – the outbreak of BSE in cattle and its association with vCJD. Although research was eventually carried out, the inception of such work was delayed – there was poor communication of the findings and, above all, conflict was evident between the interests of public health and those of industry, farming and feed production. This demonstrates very clearly the need for EPHR to be independent and able to comment on industrial (farming) practices, and the need to be open and honest in the communication of results, even if they threaten an important economic interest, and to be willing to admit ignorance when reputable findings are not yet available.

These two specific examples illustrate the important role that politics plays in EPHR. We have tried to describe the most important research in the UK and the US in three time periods. There are some general conditions that influence EPHR, and we have described these. Both the quality and quantity of EPHR has improved with time. Although the UK and US are very different in size and wealth, the general conditions of life have been similar since the end of World War I.

The type and quality of EPHR, however, has differed. Between 1918 and 1939 we consider that the relevance and quality of EPHR was greater in the US than in the UK. Both countries had similar problems – rapid industrialisation and poverty through the Depression. But there were stark contrasts. In the US the more affluent were concerned with the lot of the deprived. Most of the politically active were concerned with progress and reform while the UK had not yet come to terms with new post-war circumstances.

This influenced EPHR. While work in the US was concerned with population health, that in the UK was still more concerned with laboratory studies. The US had an organisation (the USPHS) which provided a focus for EPHR, and a specific mandate to explore and improve the health of the deprived. This was lacking in the UK. In addition the US had an academic basis, the Schools of Public Health, concerned with populations, rather than the dominant, authoritarian medical schools.

A further illustration of this was the generosity of large individual Foundations in donating substantial resources to EPHR both in the US and abroad. The US culture of enterprise – as well, of course, as its immense wealth – may be responsible for the feeling that individuals have to make their own way in the world and should not be dependent on the achievements and wealth of their parents. UK attitudes tend to value the ability to provide funds for subsequent generations.

In both countries there was industrial strife but the divisions between the different sectors of society were not so marked among the economic classes in the US compared to the UK, although, of course, the disparity and attitudes towards black people in the US did not change until the late 1960s.

The period 1945–1975 was different. The quality of EPHR in the UK was somewhat better than in the US, in spite of economic problems in the former. After World War II, UK politics and society differed radically from the period before the war. Both the main political parties were concerned with the improvement of conditions for the poor and deprived, there was a feeling of solidarity. The best manifestations of this were changes in the provision of health services (introduction of the NHS) and improvements in education. EPHR in the UK thrived – there was a feeling of great optimism, and the development of new methods of inquiry and research aimed at tackling the major causes of death and illness.

By contrast, politics and society in the US were becoming very conservative, isolationist and more involved in harvesting the material products of a consumer society. There was far more emphasis on laboratory research, and its application in the US. Some of this, of course, had important effects on health, as with, for example, polio vaccination. Fee and Brown[4] have recently suggested that in this period the development of CDC and concentration on infectious disease surveillance, with a lack of concern with chronic disease, were linked to the political fears of biological warfare. The advent, and aftermath, of the Vietnam War changed attitudes in the US and there was once again an expansion of EPHR work. In the UK the consensual politics of the 1960s were abandoned with the advent of the Conservative government under Margaret Thatcher. Gradually the climate for EPHR began to change again in the UK – and concern with the problems of deprivation and its effects on health reappeared at the end of this review period.

Recent Decline in EPHR in the UK

In the last 10 years there has been an increasing ambivalence in the attitude of the medical profession to EPHR. In the period 1945–1975 the contribution of EPHR to improved health and services was generally accepted and recognised. Now the profession (and population) are far more interested in the individual than in the population – which spills over to regard for EPHR and leads to scepticism as to what it can contribute to the health of the individual.

In the UK we have not been helped by internal schisms between the major institutions. Within London, for example, the disproportionate amount of university funding allocated to the London School of Hygiene as compared with that to the medical schools attempting to teach public health to medical students in the 1960s and 1970s led to a great deal of strife between the staffs of these institutions. This has diminished over the years but the amount of cooperation between the School and other institutions is still far less than would be expected. Similarly, within the PHLS there has always been rivalry between the demands of the laboratories in the service and those responsible for disease surveillance. Epidemiology was not regarded as an important function for many years.

The separation of environmental health from the public health function in local authorities in 1972, with public health subsequently becoming part the NHS while environmental health remained within local authorities, has undoubtedly been detrimental. EPHR has often felt inhibited from undertaking appropriate environmental research, while local authorities have been overwhelmed by service and education and so have not had the time and resources to develop appropriate research.

Since the Griffiths Report in 1983 there has been an increasing growth of managerialism in the NHS. Although this has provided major benefits to some areas of the NHS, it has often proved inhibiting to EPHR. Although good managers require and recognise the need for research, their time-scale is often so short that good medium- and long-term research cannot be undertaken and the work commissioned is superficial and inadequate. Furthermore, managers now move more frequently from job to job so that the necessary continuity of relationships is difficult to establish.

For the past 10 years, universities in the UK have been subject to what is known as the Research Assessment Exercise (RAE). This judges the research output of a University, and its Departments/Schools, on a six-point numerical scale. The highest scores are given for research of international excellence. Public health is usually grouped with other subjects such psychiatry and general practice. The difficulty of EPHR (and clinical research in general) is that it is an applied field, and the problems tackled are often of great importance and relevance locally or nationally rather than internationally. Since the judges are predominantly eminent academics and only rarely responsible for the delivery of services, EPHR does not score highly. As university funding is partly dependent on RAE grading, the funds for EPHR have not kept pace with needs, and in some places have diminished.

As mentioned above, the rewards for EPH researchers have not kept pace with those for clinicians, whose training schemes are often less complex. This has meant that the recruitment of researchers, particularly with a medical qualification, has become more difficult.

Data protection laws also have an inhibiting effect on EPHR. In the UK we have for many years lacked general or specific registers for specific diseases such as cancer or "at risk" groups. This is beginning to inhibit EPHR greatly because it is even more difficult to establish registers when this methodology is essential to answer some current questions.

The Future

It is always difficult and usually unwise to predict the future in any field of endeavour. But there are lessons to be learnt from what has gone before.

EPHR is an important area in terms of improving the health of populations and thus, ultimately, of individuals. The findings of EPHR have had an important effect on quality of life, length of life and health in the world. We have tried to analyse some of the factors which may have contributed to the quality of output at different times. There are, obviously, some factors common to all time periods and countries – adequate resources and an institutional framework enabling multidisciplinary work to be fostered, support from the professions responsible for providing a health service, and, more subtly but absolutely vital, political and societal interest and support. A clear imperative at all times is independence and freedom to enquire and disseminate findings. The need to remember that the ultimate goal of all EPHR is applied knowledge to improve health and quality of life is paramount. With increasing wealth, with increasing interdependence between groups in all parts of the world, with increasing dominance of the industrial-entrepreneurial sections of our societies and with increasing relationships between our governments and industries, there are real threats to EPHR.

The lessons of the past have shown the need for EPHR to be able to ask questions and tackle problems which may not sit comfortably with politics or industry. But there is an even greater problem. With developments in the laboratory sciences, molecular technology, mathematics, statistics and computing, EPHR is already far more interested in the analysis of micro-mechanisms and processes and far less in the solutions of macro problems such as health inequalities or ineffective health services. Investigation of mechanisms and processes is reminiscent of the preponderance of laboratory research between the wars in the UK. This is far less threatening – and far more likely to lead to immediate reward than the tackling of macro problems.

But EPHR on both sides of the Atlantic has a superlative record of achievement in improving the health of our populations. It is crucial now that it does not lose its way or compromise but continues to ask and answer the relevant and sometimes unpopular questions effectively and with scientific rigour.

REFERENCES

1   Braun D. (1994) *Health Research and its Funding.* Country Reports. Vol. I – USA and Germany. Vol. II – Great Britain and France. Bonn: Bundesministerium für Forschung und Technologie.

2   Austoker J, Bryden L (Eds). (1989) *Historical Perspectives on the Role of the MRC.* Oxford: Oxford University Press.

3   Ben-David J. (1962) Scientific productivity and academic organisation in nineteenth century medicine. In: *The Sociology of Science.* Barber B, Hirsch W (Eds). New York: The Free Press of Glencoe.

4   Fee E, Brown TM. (2001) Pre-emptive biopreparedness: can we learn anything from history? *American Journal of Public Health,* 91: 721–726.

5   Holland WW, Stewart S. (1998) *Public Health: The Vision and the Challenge.* London: Nuffield Trust.

Did Epidemiology and Public Health Research Have an Impact on Health in the Former German Democratic Republic?*

FRANK P SCHELP

The event often referred to as the "Fall of the Berlin Wall", but known by West Germans as "unification" and by East Germans as "change" divided and still divides the German population into two factions with very clear differences in feelings, perceptions and opinions.

The question under consideration in this annexe is whether EPHR had an impact on public health policy and measures in the former German Democratic Republic (GDR). Insufficient information exists to allow a straightforward answer – the question may even be irrelevant since the public health measures implemented by the authorities in the GDR were required to be in line with party and government policy. The health system was of the NHS type and the quality and efficiency of the health delivery system was the highest in the Eastern European countries. In general, throughout the whole health system and regardless of political opinions, public health issues were well understood and accepted in the GDR. But in practice this was not translated into better population health as compared to West Germany, for a number of reasons.

The West German population was considerably larger than that of East Germany and between 1950 and 1991, a slight increase was observed in the former and a slight decrease in the latter. The usual proxy health indicators for East and West Germany differed around the time of unification. Infant and maternal mortality was somewhat higher in the former GDR and male and female life expectancy lower than in West Germany.

---

* See note on page 194

Cancer incidence increased steadily when the periods between 1961–65 and 1981–85 were compared. Fewer cancer deaths, however, were reported in the GDR population in comparison with the West German population. The issue is complicated by the fact that the GDR operated a compulsory nationwide cancer registry, and coding for cancer deaths was done by medical doctors. In West Germany this was and is done by trained laymen who operate strictly according to the rules adjusted to WHO norms. In the GDR, certain population groups, such as the army, the police force and the secret service, were excluded from the reporting system. Thus it may be that the recording system there was manipulated to keep cancer deaths low. If cancer and other diseases were found in the same patient, it may also have been that death was attributed to a cause other than cancer. It is, therefore, difficult and potentially misleading to compare mortality between East and West. A detailed investigation, however, did reveal that cancer mortality was higher among the younger age groups in the East.

Mortality from cardiovascular disease could not be adequately assessed. It is therefore impossible to distinguish between East and West Germany.

Preventive medicine in relation to infectious diseases was effective because of the existence of compulsory vaccination programmes. Clear improvements were achieved in the GDR in relation to major infectious diseases, particularly TB, typhoid, viral hepatitis and measles. AIDS and HIV were practically unknown, possibly as a result of restrictions on travel, and drug addiction was uncommon.

A number of disease registries, such as the one for cancer already mentioned, and for diabetes mellitus and TB, existed. Data systems were unified and standardised in the following areas:

- Mother and child health care was well established.

- Health surveillance on pre-school and school-age children was carried out.

- Cancer screening programmes existed.

- Rehabilitation for chronic diseases existed.

- Dispensary care was offered for several diseases including diabetes mellitus, rheumatism, cardiovascular diseases and TB.

Improvements had also been achieved in occupational health and in morbidity and mortality from road traffic accidents. There was great emphasis on the health of workers who received regular check-ups. But no real population health benefit appears to have resulted from these extensive services.

EPHR was done and was needs oriented. Examples of work carried out include a study on the effect of dispensary care for rheumatism and a study to assess the efficiency of screening programmes for cervical cancer. Policy did not tend to be challenged by research but EPHR research results did lead to suggestions being made to the health authorities, and co-operation with foreign researchers was possible and did exist. Contacts with West German colleagues in the field of public health and epidemiology, however, were minimal.

The dark side of public health issues was evident. If research involved "sensitive" areas, considered either to be against the socialist ideology or to affect the image of the state, it could not be carried out or results disseminated. Data on suicides, for example, were not published for a number of years when suicides certainly occurred, especially among the older age groups.

There seemed to be no public health perspectives for the elderly, and the economic situation of those no longer of working age was not good. Retired individuals, for example, were allowed to travel to the West and to take up permanent residence there if they so wished. In contrast, the attempt to "escape" was considered a criminal offence for everyone else, with many being killed by East German border guards when trying to cross the Berlin Wall or other boundaries.

Investigations into environmental pollution – for example, studies of the use of brown coal to generate electricity or of harmful industrial production – were either stopped or results suppressed. No research was carried out in some areas – such as effects on health of social class, occupation, inequality and housing – because, according to the prevailing ideology, no problems existed in these areas.

Some important areas were explored only because of pressure from influential people involved in public health matters within the GDR. One example of this is alcoholism. When total alcohol consumption was calculated, it was found to be higher in the East than in the West, and "hard" drinks (spirits) were also more commonly consumed in the East. Mortality from cirrhosis of the liver within the 55–64 year age group was higher in the GDR than in West Germany.

The situation in relation to public health and to EPHR in the GDR can be summarised as follows:

• Preventive measures had been largely integrated into the overall health delivery system and actively implemented.

• Seen in the context of education and health development, emphasis on health was especially directed towards young children. The health of workers was also of special concern with attempts, for example, being made to forbid smoking in the workplace – a measure not finally implemented for fear of unrest.

• Although responsibility for health was seen as a task for the whole of society, it was in fact in the hands of the State and its authorities, with less emphasis on the role and responsibility of the individual.

There are many reasons why prevention in the GDR was not as effective as it might have been. Among these are the following:

• Economic restraints did not favour the active implementation of preventive measures. This was particularly true in the field of occupational medicine where old and outdated machinery as well as outdated methods of production produced occupational hazards and environmental pollution.

• In the field of nutrition, meat and milk products with reduced fat content were not always available and there was often a lack of variety of vegetables and fruit.

• Sport was not well supported as a population-based activity. The emphasis was rather on producing top athletes to support the image of the State.

• Epidemiology and health education did not work together as closely as they should have.

In general, despite all the many ideological difficulties and constraints, a generally favourable attitude to a public health approach to the management of the health of the population was present in the former GDR, one that the authorities in the West have failed to adopt and integrate into the present health delivery system in Germany. Compulsory vaccination and immunisation, for example, could have been adopted and integrated as it has been successfully elsewhere in Europe. The system of regular health checks for all workers could have been more widely introduced.

In summary of the differences in EPHR before and after the unification of Germany, two issues from the point of view of one who has seen both sides of the "Wall" stand out:

- It is now much easier for EPHR to ask the relevant questions but much more difficult to obtain the funding to research them.

- Research now may be more open but, because of the structure of the health system, answers are more elusive and there is a much reduced emphasis on prevention.

NOTE

This annexe has been produced as a result of discussions between its author and a number of researchers in the GDR who have been involved in EPHR both before and after unification. This discussion has deliberately been kept anonymous to protect the identities of the individuals.

Bovine Spongiform Encephalopathy (BSE): The first 15 years

MICHAEL O'BRIEN

In December 1984 a UK farmer called a veterinary surgeon to examine a cow that was behaving unusually. Seven weeks later the cow died. Early in 1985 more cows from the same herd developed similar clinical signs. Subsequently other herds became involved. In November 1986 Bovine Spongiform Encephalopathy (BSE) was first identified as a new disease. Later it was reported in the veterinary press as a novel progressive spongiform encephalopathy. Later still, the causal agent of BSE was recognised as an abnormal prion protein.[1]

The first few cases heralded an epidemic which at its height in 1992 gave rise to nearly 37 000 confirmed cases of BSE. Between 1988 and the end of 2000, more than 35 000 farms had been affected and a total of nearly 178 000 cattle had been confirmed as having the disease.

Control measures were first introduced in August 1988 and gradually developed until they were comprehensive and effective in 1996. In the 10 years ending 31 March 1997 the epidemic had cost the UK taxpayer nearly £300 million, almost half of which went on compensation for the farming industry. Some £61 million were spent on research.

The costs borne by the farming and associated industries are unquantified but considerable. For instance, £4 million is recorded as having been lost before compensation was introduced. Farmers also now have to pay to have fallen stock removed; previously they were paid for the carcasses. The export of cattle, beef and related products was stopped. UK consumption of beef fell, though to some extent this was offset by an increase in poultry consumption.

In 1996, despite repeated earlier reassurances about risk to human health being remote, it was accepted that a new variant of Creutzfeldt-Jakob Disease had emerged, which had affected some young people, was the same as BSE and, therefore, that it must have crossed from cattle into humans.

It was only in 1997 that a formal inquiry into the events was established by the UK government. The inquiry report has described BSE as a peculiarly British disaster.[2] Yet there is emerging evidence of its spread beyond the UK.[3,4]

Since its beginning in 1985, recognition of the significance, the scale and the control of BSE have been beset by problems (Box 1).[5] The inquiry report, though remarkably moderate in its overall tone, has confirmed this list of problems.[2]

Box 1
Problems encountered in coping with BSE
1. Delays
2. Conflict
3. Poor communication
4. Inappropriate action

All these problems are interrelated and interdependent. Delays, for example, have both stemmed from and contributed to poor communication. Conflict has contributed to both delays and inappropriate action. Inappropriate action has led to further delays, and so on. Some examples of the problems are set out in the following paragraphs.

Delays

Although The BSE Inquiry Report cites some examples of commendably prompt reaction to developments, the unfolding epidemic of BSE has been characterised by consistent and sometimes considerable delays in recognition of the significance of the new disease, in its investigation, in the provision of advice and in implementing effective control measures (Box 2).

Box 2

Delays associated with control of BSE

1. Recognition of a new disease
2. Recognition of its human health significance
3. Implementation of effective control measures
4. Start of research
5. Start of human public health surveillance
6. Coordination of effort

Nine months after the first cow was reported to the veterinary surgeon, specimens from it were referred to the Central Veterinary Laboratory for specialist opinion. A week later a diagnosis of spongiform encephalopathy was made but it was believed to be a result of exposure to a toxic substance rather than a transmissible agent. It was another 10 months before the existence of a new disease was accepted after similar pathological changes were found in animals from the first and other herds. Despite veterinary recognition of the potential impact of a new bovine disease on both commerce and human health, there was a failure to acknowledge quickly and openly its public health significance. As a consequence, it was seven months before Agriculture Ministers were advised of the existence of a new disease, and nine more months passed before the news was given to the Department of Health.[1,2,6] It was March 1988 before the Chief Medical Officer first heard of the new disease.

Veterinary epidemiology began in May 1987 and soon established a causal relationship with the use of meat and bone meal (MBM) in ruminant feedstuffs.[1,2] It was in June 1988, seven months after the causal relationship was demonstrated, that the use of MBM in ruminant feedstuffs was banned. The report cites a distinguished epidemiologist as saying that this was a "spectacularly successful control measure – one of the notable success stories of global disease control."[2] While acknowledging the benefits of hindsight, this has to be one of the most outstanding examples of hyperbole in the English language. In an equally outstanding example of understatement the report accepts that the measure was not a total success. Some of the reasons for the lack of success are discussed below, in consideration of the inappropriate actions associated with the BSE epidemic. In short, it was almost nine years before the ban was made fully effective by gradual increases in the restrictions on the use of MBM, and its extension to cover all farm animals. There was need for a parallel complete ban on the use of all offals and mechanically recovered meat (MRM) in human food. This was finally achieved in 1995, having been started in 1989.

Soon after the Department of Health was notified, but 18 months after recognition of the new disease, the first scientific working party was established to consider BSE. It was 1990, two years later, before it was changed into a dedicated Spongiform Encephalopathy Advisory Committee (SEAC) with wide terms of reference to advise the Ministry of Agriculture, Fisheries and Food (MAFF) and the Department of Health (DH). SEAC held a meeting on epidemiological methods necessary for the study of the transmission of BSE some 10 months after its establishment.

Rather more than two years passed after the first recognition of the existence of a new disease before the UK government established a committee to advise on research into the cause of BSE and its mode of spread. Although that committee produced a report after only three months, it was another six months before the government responded, citing the lack of availability of research funding to justify the delay. In other words, over three years elapsed after BSE had been accepted as a new disease before government-sponsored research finally began. By 1996–97 some £61 million had been committed to research into BSE: 52% by the Ministry of Agriculture, Fisheries and Food (MAFF), 36% by the Biotechnology and Biological Sciences Research Council (BBSRC) and comparatively little by the Department of Health (DH) and the Medical Research Council (MRC).

Although the Department of Health sponsored surveillance of Creutzfeldt-Jakob Disease (CJD) in 1990, it was 1997, 18 months after acceptance of new variant Creutzfeldt-Jakob Disease (vCJD) as a new form of human spongiform encephalopathy, that SEAC set up a subgroup to consider its epidemiology.

In short, the UK government allowed more than 10 years to elapse after recognition of the new disease before formal efforts were made to integrate the work of all the agencies concerned with the control of BSE.[1]

Conflict

From the outset, government ministers claimed that their priorities were to protect both public health and the UK farming industry simultaneously.[6,7] Thus they tried to serve two masters and failed both. The Ministry of Agriculture was faced with the dual responsibility of representing the interests of both food producers and food consumers. This produced an internal conflict of interest which led to accusations of favouring the producers at the expense of consumers. The respect of both the media and the public were forfeited at the time,[6,8] although the BSE Inquiry Report has subsequently absolved the Ministry of this failing.[2]

Within government, there was conflict between departments over "territory". The report cites examples of inadequate liaison between MAFF and the Department of Health (DH). These apparently arose because BSE was perceived, erroneously as it transpired, as an exclusively animal or veterinary issue. As such, no need was seen for either help or interference from the DH. Similarly, when the Chief Medical Officer suggested the appointment of a coordinator of research, the Research Councils and MAFF were resistant to what was seen by them as potential interference with their independence.

There has been conflict between the UK government and the European Union (EU). The latter prohibited the export of beef and beef products from the UK in 1996. The ban was not lifted until three and a half years later in August 1999, when the EU accepted that control measures were adequate and the epidemic was waning. Despite the fact that the ban had been lifted, there continued to be conflict with individual European governments because of their refusal to honour the decision of the EU and open their markets to UK beef once again. There was even threat of legal action.[9]

In the early years of the epidemic there was conflict between the government and the farming industry. The government wished the industry to bear the costs incurred by adoption of a slaughter policy. To some extent this was because of poor understanding of both the scale and thesignificance of the problem. As understanding improved, compensation was provided from public funds, firstly at a level of 50% of the value of the animals killed and later at full value.

At a professional level there were conflicts between various theories of the causation of BSE. Initially it was believed that scrapie had crossed the species barrier from sheep to cattle. Scrapie had been recognised for over 200 years but had never been recorded as affecting humans. Conventional wisdom said that humans would continue to be safe because transmissible spongiform encephalopathies (TSEs), of which BSE is one example, did not cross species barriers. The suggestion that it could have been transmitted from sheep to cattle was an apparent contradiction which was rejected for a significant time. Later, in an analogy with Kuru, it was recognised that recycling of cattle products through the MBM rendering process meant that cattle had been turned into cannibals; the infecting prions might have come originally from cattle and been concentrated before being fed to other cattle.[10,11] There was conflict about the part played in the cause or potentiation of BSE by the use of organo-phosphate insecticides in animal husbandry. Another alternative theory drew an analogy with human iatrogenic CJD by suggesting that bovine-derived growth hormones, used to boost milk yield and alter reproductive function, were the source from which prions had been concentrated by recycling through the rendering process.[12]

There have been conflicts between orthodox scientific understanding and those who have voiced unorthodox possiblities.[6] At an early stage, those who said that there might be a risk to human health were dismissed as merely speculative.[13] It has now been acknowledged that BSE has spread from cattle to humans, in the form of vCJD. It has been alleged that it might have spread through the use of vaccines containing bovine material rather than by eating infected meat.

Poor Communication

The BSE Inquiry Report [2] states that for the first six months after the recognition of a new disease, it was MAFF policy to restrict the dissemination of information on the subject. As a consequence, veterinary surgeons in practice around the country were not alerted. In particular, they were unable to relate this newly recognised disease to similar previously unrecognised cases from earlier years. A paper and letter for publication in the professional press were suppressed. It was even suggested that universities and research institutes should not be approached for help. Relaxation of the restrictions on the spread of information coincided with the beginning of veterinary epidemiological investigations.

Poor communication was not restricted either to the UK or to the veterinary world. There was delayed communication between MAFF and the Department of Health, as mentioned above. Although there were worries in MAFF about the possiblities of iatrogenic disease being caused by veterinary medicines, these concerns were not transmitted promptly to the Department of Health. There was delay in obtaining specialist neuropathological advice. Before 1990 reliance was placed on "communication with the EU and the Office International des Epizooties" instead of direct contact with countries which imported cattle and beef from the UK.

It was said that initial delay and, later, the nature of early advice to the public was aimed at avoiding panic and protecting the UK beef industry.[7] The media quoted Ministers' repeated reassurances that British beef was perfectly safe to eat. Television viewers were treated to the sight of a Government Minister trying to feed a beefburger to one of his small daughters. For several years in the late 1980s and early 1990s, advice to the public said that risks were remote. The advice was based on false assessments of the scale of the problem and false assumptions about its cause. Although it had been recognised that cattle and beef derivatives were used in the pharmaceutical and cosmetic industries and that there were potential occupational hazards for those handling cattle and bovine products, the scrapie theory of origin of the disease still held sway and caused a false sense of security. One report on risks associated with medicinal products was moderated in tone to avoid giving alarm.

Some of the reassuring advice was motivated by a wish to prevent panic and a possible failure of a public vaccination programme such as had followed alarm about pertussis vaccine a decade earlier.

There has been much debate subsequently about the meaning of the word remote. To most members of the public it meant that risks were so small as to be discounted, yet to those using the word as they offered professional advice, it meant that risks were significant but not yet defined.

In short, Government Ministers were too fond of making scientific pronouncements for which they lacked both the knowledge and the expertise, and some of the scientists were prone to putting an inappropriate political slant on their pronouncements.

Even after the scale and significance of BSE were recognised, communication about the risks and suitable precautions were slow. It took 14 months for an urgent professional guidance letter to be drafted. Guidance on occupational hazards in hospital laboratories and mortuaries took three years.

Now there are many sources of advice, especially on the World Wide Web. Some of them, including those set up by Government departments, are authoritative. Some, which were established in the early days, have ceased to be updated. They offer out-of-date information which is frankly misleading. Others have offered outlandish, unscientific and even more misleading views – for example, that BSE is the result of either imperialist or other political conspiracy.

Inappropriate Action
The inappropriate actions which took place can be characterised variously as accidental, unthinking, incompetent, deceitful and unlawful. Sometimes it was the absence of action that proved to be inappropriate.

The initial policy of delay in dissemination of information was explained on the basis of MAFF officials wishing to be sure of their facts before knowledge became widespread. All that it achieved, however, was further delay in obtaining some of the very facts of which MAFF wished to be sure, and therefore in recognising the scale of the problem and in establishing control measures.

Many of the statements made to the public were based on erroneous assumptions and were wholly inappropriate. Some, for example, concerned with causation, assumed that changes to the rendering process by which MBM was manufactured had allowed the scrapie agent to pass to cattle. Others continued to perpetuate the scrapie theory long after it was disproved.

Some of the reassurances were made in the mistaken belief that suitable safeguards – for example, exclusion of cattle with symptoms from the human food chain – were in place when in fact those safeguards had not yet been implemented. Some were given because of failure to recognise the scale and rate of spread of the disease. When the ban on use of animal protein in ruminant feed was first introduced, for instance, it was assumed to be reasonable to allow a few weeks for existing stocks to be used up because the risk that this leeway represented was low.

No priority was given to the development of a test for animal protein in feed because it was believed unlikely that anyone would ignore the ban. Later it became evident that, having been given leeway to expend old stocks, the feed and farming industries had widely ignored the ban, to the extent that some 42 000 cattle born after the ban ultimately developed BSE. The ban was ignored partly as a result of ignorance and accident, but it was also deliberately flouted. Commercial instinct prevailed over concern for public health in some mills and merchants' premises. There was cross-contamination of cattle feed with pig and poultry food between consecutive batches during the processing.

Spreading old MBM-containing feed on the land as agricultural fertiliser was permitted because it was assumed that dispersal of any BSE agent would make the dose received by grazing cattle too low to be of significance. Clearly, this was in ignorance of the small amount of prion necessary to cause BSE when taken up orally by cattle, sheep and goats.

The details of EU law inhibited the safe labelling of some cattle-derived products. Despite poor communication between MAFF and the Department of Health, the potential dangers of medicinal products for injection or implantation were recognised, at least to a certain extent. Nevertheless, stocks of vaccines were allowed to be used on children until 1992 because it was believed that the risks of avoidable death and residual disability from vaccine-preventable diseases outweighed the potential risks posed by BSE.

Liaison with the Department of Trade and Industry over the risks posed by bovine-derived cosmetics lacked urgency. There was potential for damage to the cosmetics industry because it is hard to imagine that, if the risks had been made public, those who used so-called premium grade cosmetics would have continued when they found out that these products contained bovine brain and offals which were only lightly processed. Eventually, under pressure from the EU, guidance was produced.

The failure to recall animal feed containing MBM until some three months after its use had been banned finally in 1996 can be classed as incompetent. The continued use of MBM in that three-month period was either incompetent or downright deceitful.

The slaughter of animals with symptoms, for inclusion in the human food chain, was originally, at best, unthinking. Once the connection between BSE and human disease had been established, the continuation of this practice, as was the case in some European countries, must be classed as deceitful.[14]

The final set of examples of inappropriate action surrounds the frauds that took place. There were fraudulent compensation claims. There were fraudulent attempts to show infected herds to be BSE-free. There were fraudulent schemes to present knacker meat as beef fit for human consumption in the catering and food manufacturing industries.

The Consequences of BSE
It is interesting to take stock 15 years after BSE was formally recognised as a new disease (Box 3).

Box 3
Consequences of the BSE epidemic
1. An export industry has been destroyed
2. People have been harmed
3. Experts are mistrusted
4. Government is disbelieved
5. Public health protection has been undermined
6. Anarchy has been promoted

The UK beef export industry, previously worth up to £600 million per annum, has effectively been destroyed. Despite the lifting of the European Union export embargo, some countries continued their refusal to accept British beef.[15] Home consumption of beef in the UK has declined, although this has been compensated for, to some degree, by an increase in consumption of poultry meat. The ultimate consequences for intensive farming, for the food industry, and for the price of food to consumers and for nutrition have yet to be discovered.

There is now acceptance of a causal link between BSE and vCJD, although the precise mode of spread has yet to be discovered. Up to the end of 2000, therefore, some 82 people, mainly young, have either contracted or died from a disease attributable to BSE.[16] There is no current knowledge of the scale that any vCJD epidemic might reach.

There remain further potential hazards to be faced. BSE has been transmitted to a sheep by blood transfusion.[17] The blood transfusion services take a variety of precautions, including leucodepletion of donated blood, and they import plasma from BSE-free countries. Nevertheless, although the transmission of BSE to humans by blood transfusion is unlikely, the question will not be answered definitively for a while.

There are fewer countries which can claim legitimately to be BSE-free. The World Health Organization (WHO) now reports BSE in 12 countries outside the UK.[4] So far all are in Europe but the possibility of wider transmission has been mooted.[3]

Speaking of the public, the President of the European Commission is cited as saying, "they no longer trust their governments or the scientists".[8] The BSE Inquiry provoked defensive reactions from some of the people who had to give evidence. This was understandable because there was fear that actions taken and statements made in the 1980s would be judged in the light of 1990s knowledge. Nevertheless it was a reaction which reinforced public mistrust.

It has become fashionable, in recent years, for governments to talk about concern for public health as an important factor in policy making. Unfortunately, this fashion has allowed blatant commercial protectionism, in the form of one country resisting the products of another under the guise of public health protection. This further undermines public trust and the whole concept of government-promoted public health protection.

The brief experience with public knowledge about genetically modified foods has amply reinforced the fact that confidence in expert and government statements has been lost. Instead of belief in government announcements that genetically modified foods are safe and that properly controlled experiments are being undertaken, a mixture of anarchy and sales resistance has taken over. Experimental crops have been destroyed by direct anarchic action and public attitudes have made food retailers and supermarkets withdraw genetically modified foods from sale.

BSE is not over. The possibility of its transmission to sheep through the use of MBM in ovine feed has now been recognised. Scrapie and BSE are unlikely to present differently in affected sheep. Scrapie does not spread to humans but BSE does. There must now, therefore, be critical scrutiny of sheep to ensure that they do not become another source of human disease.

Numbers of BSE cases outside the UK are growing. Cases still occur in UK cattle with 1306 cases in the year 2000. A variety of other species has been involved.[18]

Although government expenditure on the consequences of the disease has been put at £288 million by the end of 1996/7, there are predictions that controls will have to be maintained for another 15 years and that the total cost to the UK taxpayer will eventually top £4 billion.[19]

The Lessons of the BSE Epidemic

Since the introduction of quarantine to combat the spread of plague in the fifteenth century,[20] history has been full of examples of public health, commerce and politics being beset by conflict and confusion. Against this background, with its lessons derived from earlier high-profile public health problems, conflict and confusion should have been avoided when Bovine Spongiform Encephalopathy (BSE) started in the United Kingdom in 1985. It might have been expected that its significance for human health would have been recognised, communicated and researched earlier. Information to the public should have been both timely and clear. Unfortunately, this was not the case.

The lessons from the BSE experience in the UK should have been clear and simple (Box 4) and universally applicable to all countries experiencing this and other new diseases. The learning, however, has, at best, been patchy thus far.

Box 4
Lessons from the BSE epidemic

1. Allow farm animals to eat their natural food
2. Keep diseased animals out of the human food chain
3. Separate the responsibilities for commerce and public health
4. Establish public health surveillance and disease registers
5. Promote timely research
6. Tell the truth

One of the earliest recommendations to be made was to stop ruminant herbivores being fed MBM, in other words, to stop them being cannibals. The initial response was one of worry about the effect on the rendering industry. Commerce, in other words, came before public health precautions. Since June 1996, however, all farmed animals in the UK, including fish, have been protected from eating mammalian MBM. The same is not true everywhere. Quite recently mammalian MBM has still been reaching cattle in Europe, sometimes illegally labelled.[14]

A few years ago it was estimated that 200–300 animals infected with BSE still reached the human food chain in the UK annually. In the rest of Europe an unquantifiable number of infected cattle reach the human food chain, often because animals with central nervous system symptoms are sent for slaughter before diagnosis.[14] Breaches of BSE controls are still found.[21]

Many countries have long-established public health surveillance systems. The EU has agreed on a communicable diseases surveillance and control system which might eventually be connected to a global network. Such a network will have to acknowledge the part played by the WHO and complement rather than compete with it. In the meantime, the challenge will be to link existing human, microbiological and veterinary surveillance systems, both within and between states, so that relevant results in each system are readily accessible to the others. The emergence of, for example, HIV/AIDS, legionellosis and *E.Coli* O157 in the last couple of decades should have underlined the need for those responsible for surveillance to expect the unexpected and to examine unorthodox theories carefully before discarding them.

In the UK, a Food Standards Agency has been established to separate the responsibilities for producers and consumers which had been held by the Ministry of Agriculture Fisheries and Food (MAFF). Experience will show whether the new agency can change the culture and rise to the expectations of both government and the public. Other countries have their own arrangements for safeguarding the public but infected food still gets through the net. The EU may eventually have its own Food Standards organisation but the task of coordinating policies across Europe against a background of intense commercial competition between states will not be easy.

After a slow start, relevant research is now under way. One of the lessons that should be learnt is that communication of results should not be suppressed. There has for some time been argument about the ownership of research results, with sponsors claiming the right to control publication. When the sponsor is a Government department, the taxpayer is the ultimate source of the funds and, as such, has a right to know the true outcome. It is not satisfactory for a Government department or individual official to adopt a paternalistic approach and deny publication on the grounds that it might not be good for the public to know the truth. In the future there might be occasions when, to avoid unnecessary delay, scientists make public their misgivings about aspects of the management of similar problems. To do so would call for critical judgement and professional bravery when employment, career advancement and future research funding could be at stake.

Another lesson must be that experts should be more prepared to respond to questions with "I don't know" until their research produces convincing answers. It will be a difficult discipline to maintain in the competitive world of research and in face of media pressure, but they will not create panic by being truthful and could even regain the confidence of a public which is trusted to make its own choices in light of the uncertain state of the knowledge.

Similarly, politicians would be wise to acknowledge ignorance on occasions. This would require their education to a degree that ensured both understanding of epidemiological principles and insight into the effects of their pronouncements on the public.[22] Given the acknowledged loss of public confidence, it might have been expected that politicians would be more circumspect in their comments than they were at the start of the BSE epidemic. Yet, as recently as September 1999, a UK Minister of State for the Environment tried once again to serve the two masters of public health and commerce. In a BBC broadcast he said that there was no risk to human health or the environment from genetically modified oil seed rape.[23] Having given this absolute reassurance, he went on to contradict himself by speaking of the need for research in order to learn the potential impact on the environment. It is difficult to imagine how he thought members of the public could be expected to accept his initial reassurance.

The sad conclusion is that there has been conflict within and between public health, commerce and politics within and beyond the UK throughout the BSE epidemic. Despite all the clear and simple lessons, there is no evidence to suggest that such conflict and the consequential inevitable mistakes will not be repeated when new public health problems are encountered either in the UK or elsewhere. Yet there remains the ever-present hope that it will prove possible for a future generation to learn from the mistakes of the past.

REFERENCES

1 The BSE Story 1732 to 31st December 1990.
http://www.bse.org.uk/bsestory.htm

2 The BSE Inquiry Report CD-ROM. (2000) London: The Stationery Office.

3 MacKenzie D. (2001) Tomorrow the world: have contaminated feed exports
spread BSE across the globe? *New Scientist*, 16: 10–11.

4 Number of cases of BSE reported worldwide (excluding the United Kingdom).
(2001) Geneva: Office International des Epizooties.

5 O'Brien M. (2000) Have lessons been learned from the UK Bovine
Spongiform Encephalopathy (BSE) epidemic? *International Journal of
Epidemiology*, 29: 730–733.

6 Maxwell RJ. (1997) *An unplayable hand: BSE, CJD and British Government.*
London: King's Fund.

7 Waldegrave W. (2000) The BSE Inquiry/statement 299.
http://www.bse.org.uk/witness/htm/stat299.htm

8 McKee M. (1999) Trust me, I'm an expert. *European Journal of Public Health*,
9: 161–162.

9 Helm T, Johnston P. (1999) Blair warns French of court action over beef.
Daily Telegraph. 16th October.

10 Patterson WJ, Painter MJ. (1999) Bovine spongiform encephalopathy and
new variant Creutzfeldt-Jakob disease: an overview. *Commun Dis Public Health*,
2: 5–13.

11 Brown P, Bradley R. (1998) 1755 and All That: A historical primer of
transmissible spongiform encephalopathy. BMJ, 317: 1688–1692.

12 Maddocks A. (2000) The BSE Inquiry/statement 467.
http://www.bse.org.uk/witness/htm/stat 467.htm

13 Southwood R, Epstein A, Martin W, Walton J. (2000) The BSE Inquiry/
statement 483A. http://www.bse.org.uk/witness/htm/stat483A.htm

14 Mackenzie D. (2000) Secrets and lies in Europe.
www.newscientist.com/nsplus/insight/bse/secrets

15 Jones G, Brown D, Nundy J, King T. (1999) Beef war resumes as French
keep ban. *Daily Telegraph*. 11th November, cols 1–2.

16 Department of Health (2001) Monthly Creutzfeldt-Jakob Disease
Statistics. http://www.doh.gov./cjd/stats/feb01.htm

17 Houston F, Foster JD, Chong A, Hunter N, et al. (2000) Transmission of
BSE by blood transfusion in sheep. *Lancet*, 356: 999–1000.

18 Spongiform Encephalopathies in exotic species. (2001)
http://www.maff.gov.uk/animalh/bse/bse-statistics

19 Sparrow A. (1999) Mad cow disease measure cost taxpayer £4bn.
http://www.telegraph.co.uk

20 Porter R. (1997) *The Greatest Benefit to Mankind*. London: HarperCollins.

21 Beef seized in breaches of BSE controls. (2001)
http://www.bsereview.org.uk/data/

22 O'Brien JM. (1998) Epidemiological understanding: privilege for a few
or obligation for many? *Public Health*, 112: 3–6.

23 Meacher M. (1999) Interviewed on *The World at One*, BBC Radio 4,
16th September.

BSE – UK 1988–2000

Source: MAFF BSE Information. February 2001

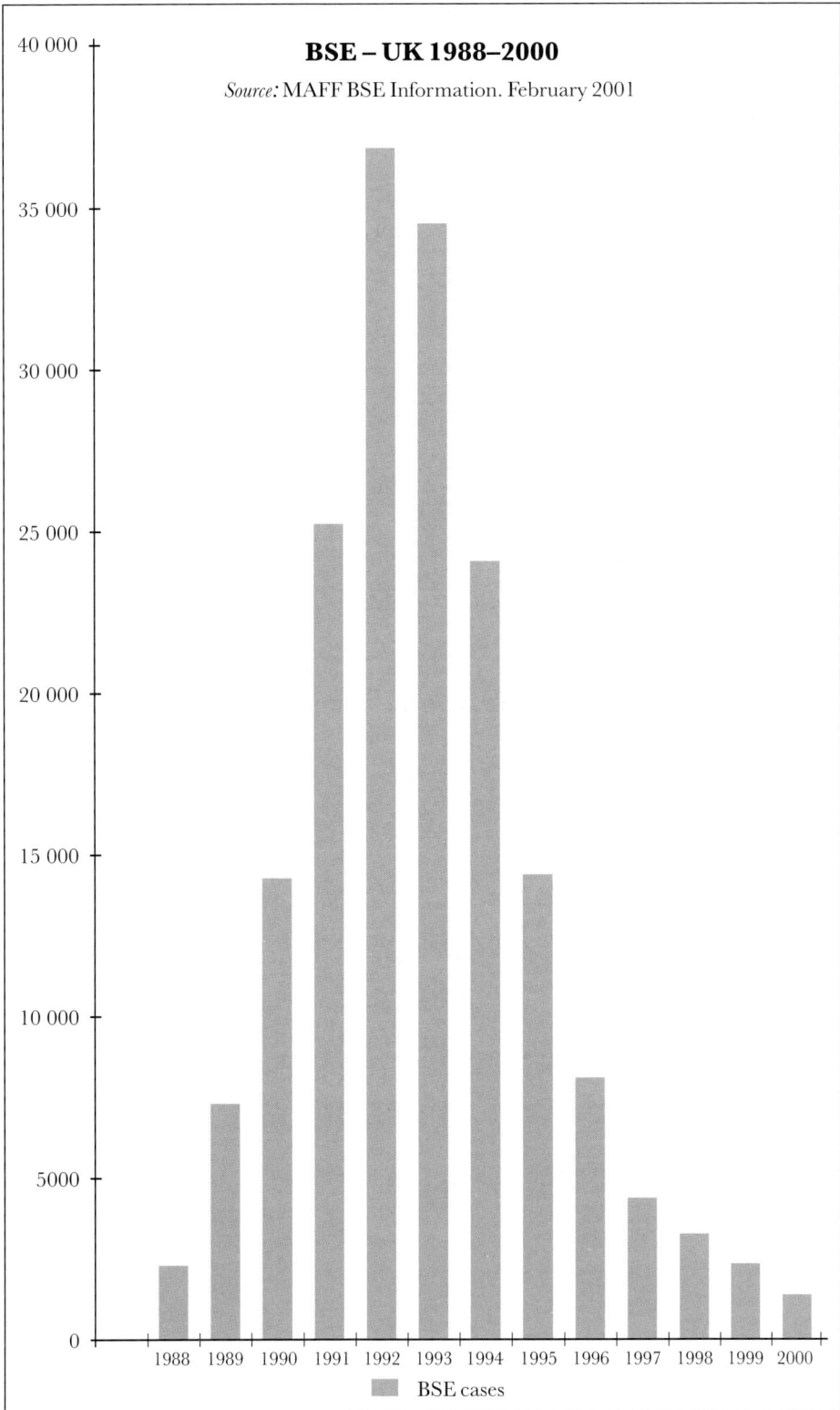

CJD/vCJD – UK 1988–2000

Source: Department of Health monthly CJD statistics. February 2001

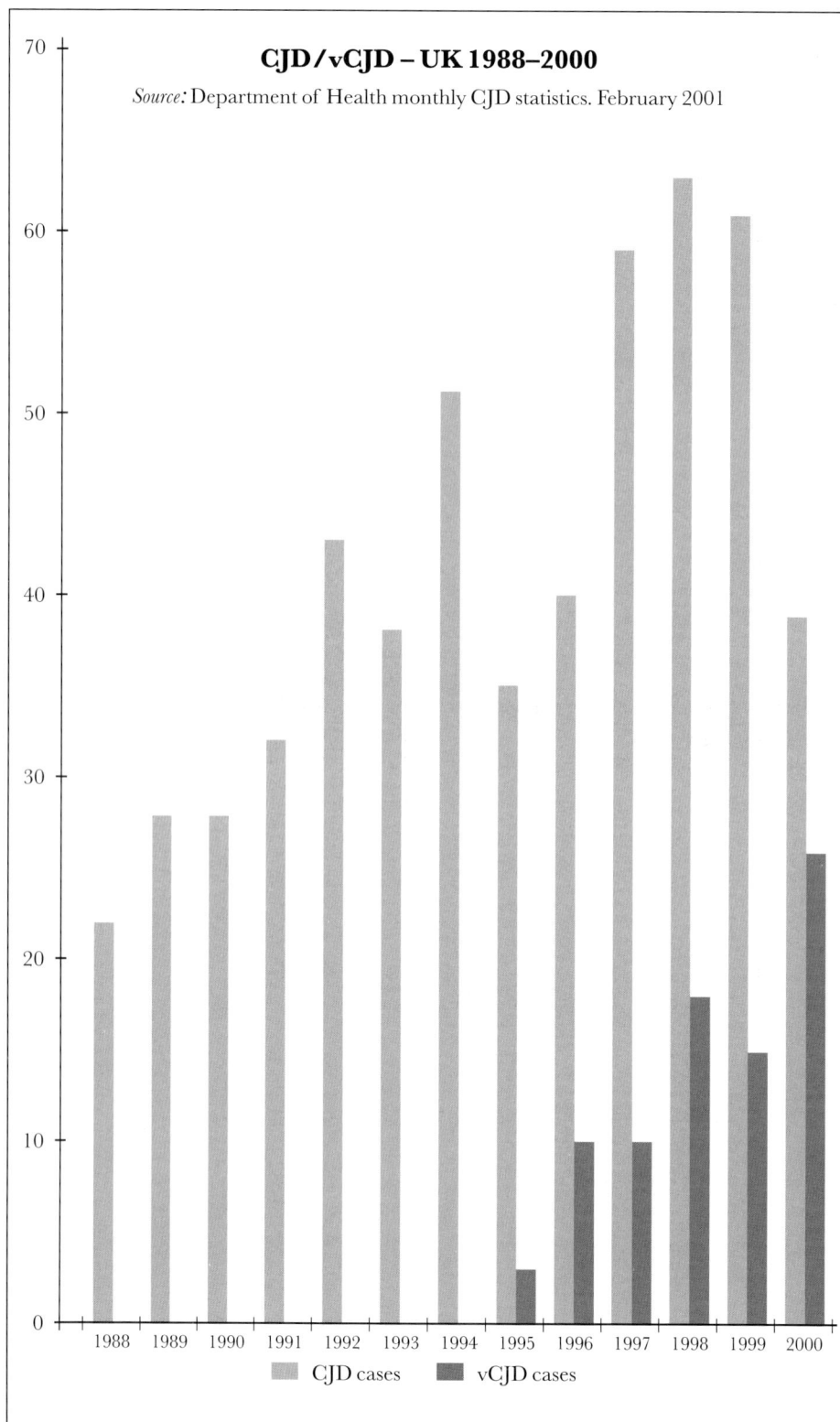

CJD cases   vCJD cases

Index